PRACTICING
AND
OTHER STORIES

PRACTICING AND OTHER STORIES

A Memoir

Ralph G. DePalma, MD, FACS

Copyright © 2005 by Ralph G. DePalma, MD, FACS.

Library of Congress Number:		2003091662
ISBN :	Hardcover	1-4134-0009-4
	Softcover	1-4134-0008-6

All rights reserved. No part of this book may be reproduced or transmitted in any form or by any means, electronic or mechanical, including photocopying, recording, or by any information storage and retrieval system, without permission in writing from the copyright owner.

This book was printed in the United States of America.

To order additional copies of this book, contact:
Xlibris Corporation
1-888-795-4274
www.Xlibris.com
Orders@Xlibris.com

CONTENTS

FOREWORD 9
PRACTICING 13
LOOKING INTO PAST LIGHT 30
RAT RACES 46
THE LION THAT BARKED 55
MEDICINE, THE MISTRESS 72
WHAT I DID ON MY VACATION 93
SEVILLENAS: AN AUDITION 108
JOURNEY TO THE WESTERN RESERVE 129
AN EASY LIFE: CLEVELAND CASES 139
RNO-ORD 158
WASHINGTON YEARS: HIGH HOPES AND
    PARTISAN POLITICS 178
RIYADH TO RENO 203
A LIFE OF THE MIND 212
SEX AND THE SURGEON 240
A VEXING PROBLEM:UNFINISHED BUSINESS 245
REFERENCES 253
CARING FOR THE GREATEST GENERATION 265

Dedicated to my parents,
Frank and Mary,
to the DeFelittas,
and to all my teachers.

FOREWORD

Surgeons tend to call attention to themselves, though individually, they may be quiet and even retiring. They possess the confidence needed to take up a knife to cure illness, and are usually certain in their actions. They must be, as surgical interventions directly connect physicians with outcomes, usually good or occasionally bad. While this can be stressful, I am content with how rewarding my work has proved to be. These are the memoirs of a surgeon who lived and worked in lively and rapidly changing times: the last half of the twentieth and the beginning of the twenty-first centuries. The unique tenor of these times shaped my life and work.

Two years before I was born in the Bronx, in New York City, the United States suffered a severe financial crisis. I grew up during that time, though, we, in New York, suffered less than the rest of the nation. The world of my childhood was a conservative yet boisterous environment, and while we labored under financial privation, great generosity also existed. My parents, first-generation Italian immigrants, carried with them Old World attitudes and behaviors. As children, many of us tried to escape this heritage, but some of it stuck. I am now grateful for this. Bonfires burned on election night and crowds around them chanted, "Roosevelt, Roosevelt, Roosevelt!" signaling the beginning of the New Deal. This gesture of *noblesse obliges* by a generous New York aristocracy saved people in my class from abject poverty, and offered opportunities never imagined in Europe. New York City and its educational system afforded us splendid opportunity. I never imagined, as a child, that I would become a physician, much less a surgeon, and that I would have the privilege to lead or to teach. I matured in turbulent times and served in the military during the threat of nuclear annihilation.

Three revolutions occurred during my life: societal, sexual, and medical. Growing up in the Bronx, I had much to learn about proper behavior. But beneficent, generous influences in New York helped to cultivate whatever was good in my character. The willingness of the establishment to overlook class distinctions, at least, in some degree, characterized that society. My flaws and faults are mainly my own. Columbia College changed my life and developed my mind; New York University School of Medicine provided me a classic professional education and a lifelong vocation.

During my lifetime, sexual behavior changed from the rigid mores of the 'thirties, 'forties and 'fifties to the sexual revolution of the 'sixties and 'seventies. We became more vulnerable but somehow more human and gentler than we had been. Sexual conservatism returned in the mid-1980s. In early 1982, a penalty for promiscuity took the form of an obscure retrovirus from central Africa that had never been seen before. The AIDS epidemic began. Sexuality forms an important part of life, and is usually not a part of a professional memoir. But it is important, so I include anecdotes, with names changed to protect the innocent. These tangential observations reveal attitudes unique to changing times, persons and places.

My generation of surgeons participated in spectacular advances made possible by our immediate predecessors. Truly, we stood on the shoulders of giants. Just as I finished surgical training in 1964, the disciplines of cardiac and vascular surgery bloomed in Cleveland, Ohio; Houston, Texas; Minneapolis, Minnesota and in a few other places. Vascular disease became my life-long interest, although other clinical and scientific challenges tempted or distracted me. Contributions in organ transplantation, intravenous nutrition, and advances in intensive care revolutionized medicine. I tried, in fact I felt compelled, to contribute to this progress in some small way.

I had the privilege of serving in leadership positions at three universities: as a professor at Case Western Reserve University and of occupying two chairs of surgery, one in Nevada and one at George Washington University. I achieved only modest national or organizational prominence, and was never elected to the pinnacle of our most important societies. I had, as a result of my early upbringing, a wish for personal anonymity; later, in midlife—a desire to clarify certain truths and relationships for myself, and only much later in life, the desire to seek to guide or influence others. The fallibility and vulnerability of leaders astonished me; leaders, even in surgery, could be quite wrong, do considerable damage and yet, continue to be perceived as leaders. So I kept myself deliberately naïve: tough on myself and sometimes too tough on others. The reader will find lessons in my doubts and errors, but, I hope, also comfort. I stumbled and wasted precious time, but many fine things happened along the way.

A wise lady once asked me what I was looking for in life. Immediately, without thinking, I replied, "The Grail." I am not sure why this came to mind, but these words came immediately to my lips. I have never grasped this cup, but I have been tantalizingly close at times, particularly when caring for patients or experiencing an insight into scientific truth. I think about how much more remains to be done in these searches. Continual change affects my life and my work, and I am still, in one way or another, practicing.

PRACTICING

> Having everything in order for what is to be done, know what you must do before going in.
> Hippocrates, *Decorum*

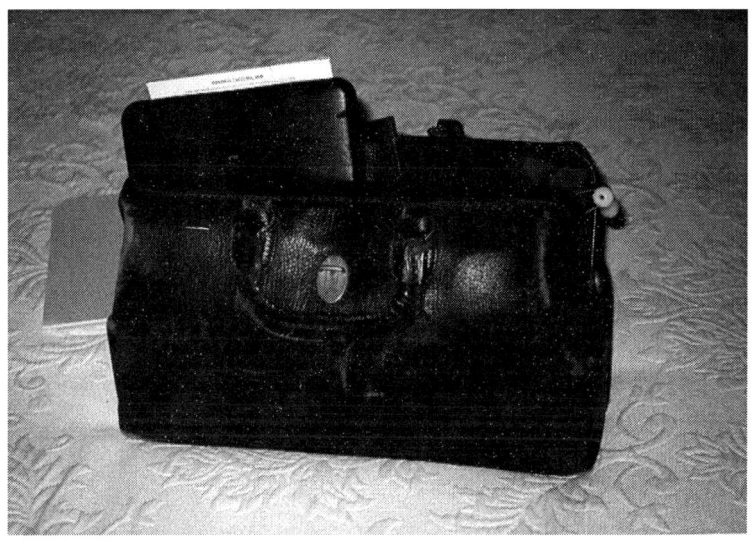

Black Bag courtesy of Merck and Company

A long time ago, the black bag was an emblem of what was to become my profession. I have a vivid recollection of the black bag carried by our family's general practitioner, Dr. Gerald Carroll, when he came to our apartment in the Bronx. A serious, quiet Irishman, Dr. Carroll had delivered me at home on East 225th Street and later cared for our family's illnesses for two decades. After we moved from the Bronx to Yonkers, he continued his house calls, driving several miles north to our new home on Kimball Avenue. He would get out of his car carrying that black bag, and we had faith that curative magic, even miracles, would emerge from its depths. Through all the years I knew him, and even after

I aspired to become a physician, I never believed I could be as good a man or as fine a doctor as Dr. Gerard Carroll. He wore horn-rimmed glasses, magnifying dark blue eyes, which focused intently on the patient. He said little, always listening more than speaking. His only known vices were Friday night poker games and chain smoking. I was in my second year of medical school at New York University when this admirable man died at fifty-five years of age. I wondered what happened to his black bag. I know that he was deeply disappointed when his son was not accepted for medical school; at that time, only one out of five applicants was taken. He appeared tired and mentioned his son sadly when I saw him for a physical examination required by my acceptance to New York University School of Medicine. "Fine," he said, brightening up, "Bellevue!" He regarded me appraisingly with serious magnified eyes.

Traditionally, the Merck Pharmaceutical Company gave each new medical graduate a black bag, and I still have mine. Hours were spent stocking them, agonizing over drugs and what instruments we might need to treat anything or everything. We believed that this was, somehow, expected. Later, in the 1970s, a time when our society was dealing with its conscience over the Vietnam War, protests were the norm. New medical graduates cynically dubbed the black bags as drug company bribes and burned them in protest. But these were fine bags and I kept mine and still have it half a century later. However, for eighteen months after graduation, during my surgical residency, the fine leather bag remained neglected, gathering dust in a hall closet.

Residency in surgery was an unbelievably hectic time at a busy New York Hospital. As interns and residents, we worked every other night, all day and on alternate weekends. For this, we received $50 a month. During my internship, there were no vacations. But no one complained. We felt privileged to have been chosen for an elite program. We even said, half jokingly, "The problem with being on every other night is that you miss half the good cases." The statement was hypocritical. Actually, most preferred an every-third-night rotation. In the last part of my second year, I was rotating on pathology only every fifth night. At the same time, I was also called, drafted really, to serve in the air force starting in August of 1958.

My wife, Eve, and I had been married for three years. We rented a bright one-room apartment on Bronx River Road in Yonkers near McLean Avenue, a bedroom suburb north of Manhattan and just yards past the northern border of the Bronx. I had grown up a few miles from here. The neighborhood was a largely Irish and Italian ethnic enclave. The mind-set of the people living in that area resembled the Queen's neighborhood of TV's *Archie Bunker*. As a young people, we attended mass each Sunday, going to confession on Saturdays and taking communion once a month. No one we knew was divorced or received welfare. People were expected to work and pay their way; we always put our money on the bar before ordering a drink. I still have certain blue-collar habits, and find it difficult to run a tab at a bar. Even worse, from time to time, I have been chided for echoing, however mildly, Archie Bunker. Such bad past attitudes are hard to outgrow and pop up like evil hobgoblins when least expected. My wife, nee Tankard, had grown up in New Jersey and we spent alternate Sunday afternoons at my mother's house on Kimball Avenue, enjoying traditional Italian Sunday dinners. My wife, characterized by some of the family as an "American Girl," liked hearty, comforting Italian food and even achieved reasonable culinary success cooking it for our own family.

One Sunday afternoon, Dr. Andrew Shilero, my mother's general practitioner, called to ask if I might cover his practice on weekends. As the pathology rotation now permitted a reasonable schedule, I considered this interesting offer. My chief resident at St. Luke's Hospital, Dr. Clayton DeWitt, encouraged me. He had done such moonlighting and suggested that I could learn from it. With a now relatively undemanding fifth-night rotation and with Clay's reassuring words, I agreed. The black bag was dusted off and stocked with injectables and syringes, batteries for the ophthalmoscope-otoscope and other carefully chosen items. Armed with my bag and a malpractice insurance policy purchased for $150 from Lloyds of London, I began this general practice.

Weekend calls came promptly; house calls in the North Bronx, Mt. Vernon and Yonkers were customary and expected. Suit and tie for house calls and relatively formal dress for all occasions were strictly observed. As one of my mentors said, "It's hard enough to be a doctor, even if you look like one." I always dressed, or at least tried to dress, the part. In the beginning, I wore a black pinstriped suit, more appropriate for a much older man, a white shirt and a rep striped necktie, a gift from my fraternity brothers at Columbia. I was twenty-five years old as I began practice, and was actually paid for my efforts. I began with trepidation. I found it gratifying to be received, at my stage of development, with awe, and at the same time, I was uncomfortable to be the undeserving recipient of the respect accorded to "the doctor."

Almost always, in each home, clean towels had been prearranged in a spotless bathroom. However modest, these households usually appeared preternaturally orderly, including the sickroom. Patients were clad in immaculate underwear or nightdress, usually pressed. The doctor's visit was a ritual meticulously prepared for well in advance. This sometimes included an ethnic hospitality, which made the need to eat regular meals unnecessary. After the history of the illness was obtained, physical examination completed, and prescriptions carefully written, food was usually offered. This might include coffee, antipasto and, on Sunday, cannoli, delicious cream-filled Italian pastries. A ten-dollar bill conspicuously displayed on the dresser was payment for services rendered. Important questions required judicious answers, "How long will it take me to get back to work, Doc?" "When can the kid go back to school?" "Should my mom come over?" "Do you think I should have my mother-in-law come in?" These house calls were a privilege for me, although, most of the time, the medical problems were simple and self-limiting illnesses in comparison to the surgical challenges of my later career. However, complacency was always a danger.

Shortly after beginning this practice, I was called at midnight to a modest apartment in Sherwood Park on Yonkers Avenue to see an eighteen-month-old with fever and vomiting. In anticipation, I had placed in my bag a vial containing penicillin, which had been stored in the refrigerator. At that time, we had nonlocking small syringes and separate needles—prepackaged syringes were a thing of the future. A touchingly vulnerable, distraught young woman answered the door with her infant in her arms. She was alone with the child. Her family lived far away in upstate New York and her husband was gone on business. The baby looked critically ill, as children with a high fever do. Rectal temperature was 105.4 degrees. To my relief, examination showed a beefy-red pharyngitis with purulent spots punctuating massively swollen tonsils. The lungs were clear. Penicillin was clearly indicated, and I carefully prepared the injection.

The young mother was obviously frightened by how sick the child looked, and so was I. Instructing her to hold the baby over her shoulder, I punctured the baby's exposed buttock in the upper, outer quadrant. The baby screamed and squirmed suddenly, and, at the same time, the mother lost her grasp. The penicillin syringe disconnected from the needle, white liquid splashed over my black suit and necktie, while the needle lodged in the tiny buttock oscillated back and forth. Trying to appear calm, I fished out of my bag another needle and empty syringe, drew more thick penicillin, still cold, from the vial, removed that needle and firmly reconnected the syringe with the oscillating needle in the child's buttock. I then injected the penicillin without event. The young woman endured this performance with surprising composure. But, by now, the child appeared worse: lethargic and almost comatose. His temperature had increased to 106 degrees.

To lower the alarming fever, I suggested a sponge bath, as I recalled receiving one from my mother, supervised by Dr. Carroll, during a bout with measles. The young woman looked puzzled; she did not know how to do this and, really, neither did I. We were not taught in medical school how to give sponge baths or intramuscular penicillin injections. I had never watched, with any attention, this procedure being done. Nurses knew all about sponge baths and injections. At 2:00 A.M., I called a friend, the duty operating room supervisor, at St. Luke's Hospital, for explicit instructions about alcohol sponges.

There was a long silence, then, I heard shared laughter. I had ordered many but, as I told the senior duty nurse, I had never done this procedure. They wanted clinical details: where was I and why? I was sweating heavily by the time the nurse instructed me, step by step, how to give a sponge bath. I was warned not to attempt to drop the temperature too rapidly. First, one extremity was sponged and exposed to the air with the others covered and the body only partly exposed. By 4:00 A.M., the temperature abruptly fell. I have been told of immersion of the entire child in cold water but I shudder, still, to think of having done that that in this case. During this time, the exhausted mother dozed in a chair. By 5:00 A.M., the baby sat up and laughed. Sick children also tend to get well rapidly. I stayed another hour to assure myself that the fever was gone and left at dawn with my spotted black suit and a sense of vast humility. I also later endured a razzing from the operating room nurses when I told the story.

Telephone conversations describing illness can be misleading. I never ask many questions when called about an acutely ill patient—it is better to go to see the patient whenever possible. One Sunday evening, I visited an upscale apartment in Bronxville to see a woman who called with vague and unspecified complaints. Her husband came on the line and firmly requested a house call, refusing to give further details. I found an apathetic young woman who spoke little and moved less. They told me that two nights before, Dr. Joseph Caricchi had seen her three-year-old girl and diagnosed bronchiolitis. The child had been given antibiotics and though she appeared to be improving, shortly after midnight, the baby suddenly died. I examined the mother, listened to her for a good while and prescribed Equanil along with a mild barbiturate for sleep. They thanked me quietly. The young woman appeared comforted by the attention even though the medications I prescribed were incorrect for treating depression. But these were the best, with the limited knowledge I could think of, and were about all the psychotropic drugs available at the time.

Clearly, the visit was more important than the medication prescribed.

The physicians' group had a kind of "rounds" every Wednesday afternoon in a relatively empty Mt. Vernon bowling alley. Here, between bowling frames, the practitioners discussed problem cases. Their comments were more critical and direct than were university morbidity and mortality conferences. The death of this child was considered in detail. All were profoundly disturbed by this death, and the doctor who made the call was devastated. In retrospect, the group felt that the doctor's response to the call had been prompt and that proper antibiotics had been administered. The autopsy did not show consolidating pneumonia that might have been detected with the stethoscope, but rather, a deceptively mild and patchy bronchopneumonia. At that time, and now once again, it was uncommon to hospitalize children for bronchiolitis. Retrospectively, all the doctors wished this had been done. Later, in an air force hospital, I saw a similar death involving an infant who had been sent home from triage by an experienced nurse practitioner after receiving antibiotics. Nurses had been assigned to triage because the doctors felt overburdened by a third-night-call schedule and emergency visits for what appeared to be trivial conditions. We immediately terminated that arrangement. Patterns of illness, like bad dreams, tend to repeat themselves over and over. Childhood respiratory illnesses, which might be regarded as simple, are in my opinion, terrifying and unpredictable.

During these sessions, I was expected to bowl. Even though I did not like to bowl and still do not, I learned a great deal of medicine on Wednesday afternoons, as my bowling score improved from the low 90s to about 150. I never did learn golf since these doctors, in that time and place, preferred bowling, even in the summer. Perhaps, these practitioners, much like their blue-collar patients, had yet to evolve to country club status. They did have strict rules, however. Promptness for the bowling sessions was mandatory. Having to drive to Mt. Vernon from

Manhattan, I was sometimes late. Whenever I was late, my 1957 Ford would have to be parked at the end of a long line of Cadillacs and Oldsmobiles. My tardy entrance was greeted with fifteen minutes of grumpy silence until it could be ascertained into which "frame" each of us was to be on the scorecard. The group did get to approve of me and several suggested that I give up surgical residency and join their practice. Well-meaning relatives also pressured me, "When are you going to stop being an intern and be a real doctor?" While still learning and enjoying my surgical craft, at $50 a month, I did not feel much like a real adult or a valued doctor. This sort of questioning was demoralizing. The group was a source of mutual support. While I was invited to expand coverage for more practitioners, one of them was always available by phone as a senior consultant. These Bronx doctors were vocal, explicit, and passionate individuals, and contrasted sharply with the remote and reserved Manhattan physicians I encountered during medical school and residency.

I was called one Saturday afternoon to an Italian funeral home because a woman had fainted. The callers resisted my well-intentioned phone instructions, which included breathing into a paper bag, smelling salts and elevation of the lower extremities. They pled, "Doc, you goatta come." As soon as I entered the crowded funeral parlor, two more women immediately fainted. Although I knew that this was a form of hysteria, I really did not know what to do. All three women stretched out on the plush carpet were heavily corseted and each exhibited deep breathing and slow pulse rate characteristic of vasovagal reactions, their faces flushed and eyes rolled upward. I called Dr. D' Angelo, who was the primary practitioner for most of this group. "What do I do about this?" "Well, Ralph, have you any Thorazine in your bag?" I quickly looked and luckily, there it was. "Well, give them each a shot, twenty milligrams IM. Charge forty dollars an injection. It will be a good afternoon for you." Actually, the Thorazine, the "shot," or both, quickly brought all three around immediately.

Respectful men in black suits and ties walked with me slowly to the door.

Technical medicine and refined diagnostics were not strong points of practice in the North Bronx precincts. I was called to East 216th Street near Bronxwood Avenue, directly across the street from our previous home. A fragile eighty-five-year-old woman, "Nona" Martucci, was falling, particularly at night, and according to her family, she had become increasingly confused. She looked quite white, exhibiting an almost translucent pallor. My black bag contained a hemocytometer and a hemoglobin meter. As Bellevue medical students, we were required to perform blood counts on our hospital patients. We had all purchased our own instruments. The hemoglobin meter showed severe anemia on the spot. I obtained a blood sample and slide to take home to my microscope for a blood count. The slide and the count showed macrocytosis, extremely enlarged red cells, a finding confirmed early the next morning by one of my resident colleagues in hematology. When I returned to Nona Martucci the next day, my bag now contained a tuning fork. She had a complete lack of vibratory sensation along with loss of position sense in her toes and feet. I had, I felt, made a brilliant diagnosis of subacute combined neurological degeneration due to pernicious anemia. I called Dr. Carletti to let him know of this triumph. This was an eminently treatable neurological condition with a good prognosis, something not often found in the elderly.

At the following Wednesday's bowling rounds, nothing was said about my diagnostic coup. I finally asked, "Well, how's Grandma Martucci getting along?" "Oh, well, she's much better," replied Carletti rather casually. "What did the bone marrow show?" I asked. "What bone marrow?" Carletti answered. "Well, you know, if she had subacute combined, we want to know what the cellular abnormalities were in the bone marrow." "Was she treated with B12 injections?" They all turned and grinned at me. Carletti slowly told me, "Well, Ralph, we gave her some Hemantamynic." "What is that?" He answered: "Well, everything, like folic acid, B12, iron, vitamin C and other stuff." I persisted, "Why didn't you do a bone marrow?" The response was incredulous: "One time, some fancy hematology guy up at New Rochelle Hospital talked us into doing a marrow on an old lady. He perforated the sternum along with the pulmonary artery. She died. Nona and her family are very happy. Why do you wanna spoil the case, she's getting better with Hemantamynic." Their lesson about the art of medicine versus the discipline of scientific medicine was that the enemy of good is better. A bone marrow would have more precisely nailed down the diagnosis and treatment. They preferred shotguns to rifles

Another provocative idea of these practitioners was that patients with ulcer disease or gastric upsets needed a "good shot of penicillin." Four decades later, we learn that most ulcers are related to a more or less penicillin-sensitive organism called *Helicobacter pylori*. When I remonstrated about the penicillin added to conventional antacid therapy, some of them laughed at me. Shoulders were shrugged upward with arms downward extended in that characteristic Italian way. "Well, it works! Try it. You'll see."

The income from this practice got progressively better. Pressure continued for me to quit the surgical residency and join their group. Luckily, I had the excuse that military service was to claim me after my resident duties ended on June 30. But I was not to escape easily. When Dr. Shilero went on vacation, he asked me to act as locum tenens at his office until August, when I was to report to the Air Force "Charm" School in Montgomery, Alabama. The financial arrangements were that half of the office fees would go to the support of his office and nurse. I was to keep for myself the house call fees of about ten dollars a visit. The income was good and the arrangement both practical and fair. I was admonished to keep exact records of collections and expenses for the IRS. I do not recall ever having to bill for a house call; cash was always on the dresser. Most office charges were also paid at the time of the visit; the nurse billed only a small proportion of these fees. Thus, I continued with my practice, learning lessons about efficiency and cost effectiveness, which helped later in an academic group practice.

Without insurance forms or the requirement to squabble with HMOs, no need existed for an elaborate office clerical staff. More importantly, I learned was how to recognize serious, real illness and how to deal effectively with a chief complaint, or at least, the patient's major concern.

Patients seemed to know, and they often still do, exactly what they needed; all the doctor had to do was ask. A cohort of attractive middle-aged ladies called at the office for their "Fem Glan injection." They pointed to the ornate glass doors in the examining room cabinet where vials labeled Fem Glan were stored. A small card for each patient indicated 1-2 cc biweekly doses as needed of "Fem Glan PRN." This practice was also far ahead of its time, as hormone supplements are now considered important in relieving distressing menopausal symptoms. Each office record was handily available on 5 X 7 file cards; as I later found, these condensed records were used in the surgical practice at Case Western Reserve. These condensed lists are more effective than a huge file and the data overload of conventional handwritten paper records. Notes were simple: "probable step infection," "penicillin 600,000 units IM," or "I and D of abscess of finger." More complex interventions were sequentially recorded along with the result, details to be found in separate files.

Just as I was becoming more confident in my judgments, a frightening episode occurred. A call came at eight o'clock on Saturday morning from another anxious mother whose husband was out of town. She had obviously waited until morning to call about her sick child. In the background, I could hear the characteristic inspiratory crow of croup. She did not feel that I needed to come to the house nor, without a car, was she able to bring the baby to the nearby office. She wanted advice. I gave her instructions about humidification, recommending either an office visit or a house call, but advising her, in any event, to call again. Two hours later, she called back. Now in the background, I heard the alarmingly high-pitched respiratory stridor of impending laryngeal obstruction. The local hospital was not that close to her home in the East Bronx. I instructed her to call an ambulance but she seemed paralyzed by fear. I drove rapidly to the neighborhood, finding a two-year-old girl in severe distress, with deep cyanosis and labored respirations. I realized with panic that my black bag did not have a tracheostomy set, but it did contain an injectable steroid, which I immediately used. While preparing the syringe, I again asked the mother to call an ambulance. She was so distraught she could not manage to dial the rotary phone. I made a quick call to an ear, nose and throat consultant in Yonkers. Then, with the mother still in her pajamas and the baby wrapped in a blanket snatched from her crib, I took them downstairs and we sped to St. Joseph's Hospital in my 1957 Ford Fairlane. The consultant was waiting and the child was placed in a humidified oxygen tent. Thankfully, the little girl's breathing improved. We stood ready to perform a tracheostomy, but, as her airway improved within the hour, the consultant felt that the steroid injection, humidification and oxygen had been sufficient. He was most gracious. We stayed until it was clear that the child was out of danger.

I had been lucky. At the next bowling session, I was told that people, particularly the family, were pleased with my actions. I was, however, admonished by my colleagues about the risk of transporting that sick child to the hospital in my personal car. I was made aware of my potential vulnerability in this situation. I learned that compromises, coupled with understandable forms of patient noncompliance, could become quite dangerous. Sometimes, problems take the form of stubborn pride. A phone call the next weekend reinforced the negative vibes of the last weekend. The service operator called on Saturday describing a man with either severe angina or myocardial infarction. The family, over the phone, insisted on an Italian-speaking doctor. I told the answering service that I did not speak Italian but spoke directly with the family. Still, the patient insisted on a doctor who could speak Italian. I gave explicit instructions to take the patient to a hospital and I asked to be allowed, at least, to examine him. The family and the patient refused. Later that afternoon, this man died. There were recriminations and the threat of a suit. Absolution came in the form of testimony of the answering service operators. The operators had listened to our telephone conversations. Their physician bluntly told the family that legal action was inappropriate. I was left wishing that I had learned to speak Italian, as my family had desired. Later, I became fluent in Spanish, which was of considerable help in treating patients in New York.

Vexing problems usually surfaced late on Sundays, after large family gatherings. One Sunday evening, I was called to the South Bronx, near the Whitestone Bridge, to see a Lebanese grandfather from Queens who was visiting his daughter and the in-laws' extended family. The crusty old man experienced a sudden onset of severe abdominal pain after eating a large meal. Physical examination was characteristic of a perforated ulcer: maximal epigastric tenderness and rebound and an abdomen rigid as a board. I contacted a surgeon at the Cross County Hospital and made arrangements to send the patient there. He refused. He wanted to go just across the Whitestone Bridge to a hospital in Kew Gardens, Queens. Intimidating the family and a young doctor, he insisted on this course of action. I foolishly gave him an injection of Demerol and Atropine, warning him that though he would feel better, he was to go directly to the hospital in Queens. We gingerly placed him, bundled in a blanket, in the back seat of his large black Cadillac. He felt and looked better. The in-laws, relieved to see him go, served Turkish coffee and baklava. At midnight, I went home to the sleep of the righteous.

Later, I got several new patient calls to this Lebanese neighborhood. "Oh, you are that young doctor who advised Mr. Katchadurian to go to the hospital. You know, he almost died." I was shocked. "We heard that you are really a good doctor even though you are young. He talked those silly women into taking him home rather than going to the hospital in Queens." In fact, he did not report to the hospital for two whole days. Though he eventually recovered, Mr. Katchadurian teetered on the brink of death after a delayed operation for perforated ulcer. I learned more about the need for persuasion in cases of serious illness. At the same time, I learned that close-knit communities have their own forms of outcome research, a sense of intrinsic fairness, and the ability to recognize stupidity.

The need to compromise with stubborn people from the old country was again learned when I was called one Sunday night to the home of the head of Cavoli Construction Company, a large establishment in the North Bronx near Paulding Avenue. An army of relatives had gathered for dinner. The stout old patriarch had recently been discharged from the hospital following a prostate operation. He was in a terrible mood. His massively swollen leg was propped up on an ottoman as he complained of pleuritic chest pain. Casual observation revealed his wracking painful coughs; he was spitting blood-tinged sputum into a grimy handkerchief. A leathery pleural friction rub was heard where he said his chest hurt. A diagnosis of pulmonary embolism could not have been more clear. With great concern I announced to him and his retinue that he must immediately return to the hospital. The old man looked me up and down for a while with scornful dark eyes. "Fukkadahospital," he said, turning his head away. I tried to reason, but nobody was going to contradict the boss of Cavoli Construction. I told him that he might die.

I called my resource backup. He listened to the story and thought about it for a while. "Why don't you give him some heparin?" he advised cautiously. "What about clotting times, and the risks?" I asked hesitantly. "Well, if you don't give him heparin, he is going to die. I know that old man; he won't go to the hospital. Besides, his son-in-law is a diabetic. He will know how to give injections." The local pharmacy delivered the heparin to the house. Wishing I were elsewhere, I injected 5,000 units intravenously and instructed the family to give 5,000 units subcutaneously at four-hour intervals. I slept poorly that night. It was with a sense of dread that next Sunday that I got a call to go back to the house. "Mr. Cavoli wants to see you." Mr. Cavoli's cheeks were now red. He now appeared in robust good health. He was drinking Campari and smoking a De Nobili cheroot. He pronounced me a great doctor "even if he is 'wet behind the ears' kid." This case would not have turned out so well had Mr. Cavoli, with his particular connections, done poorly. But I had learned more about the need to compromise when compromise was required.

We were expected to enter the home of an agitated individual suffering from acute pulmonary edema and to control the situation on the spot. In addition to a morphine injection, which yielded an immediate calming effect, my cardiology GP mentor advocated the use of intravenous rapid-acting digitalis, "Sqill," a potent drug to be given with a finger on the pulse. This was done without benefit of a monitor or knowledge of electrolyte values, but if the heartbeat became at all irregular, the injection was stopped. We then had no rapid-acting diuretics such as furosemide. Intramuscular injections of mercuhydrin, in addition to rotating tourniquets, were used to overcome the lethal fluid overload. Due to the lack of potent diuretics at that time, low potassium levels were probably relatively uncommon. Giving the digitalis preparation in the presence of low potassium would have been more frequently lethal. Delivery of an oxygen tent to the home was prompt. After an hour or two of sitting by the bedside and listening to the lungs of the patient, one could hear the deadly pulmonary tide turning. A resting patient and a relieved family were ample rewards. We had yet to invent intensive care units, and now, I wonder what pulmonary catheter pressure readings and continuous EKG monitors might have shown. But one thing we learned was the ability to recognize a critically ill person and to treat on clinical grounds, and without delay. The treatment of those times was not optimal. My own father died when I was nine as a result of pulmonary edema that began in the middle of the night, but then, he was taken to the hospital, as Dr. Carroll was somehow unavailable or not called.

The privilege of treating people is something precious and doing so in their homes, even more precious. The general practitioner, William Carlos Williams, also a poet, wrote: "They called me and I came." This was a lesson never forgotten in my life as a physician and, then, as a surgical specialist. When called, you must see the patient. Only in the direct encounter will the doctor learn what needs to be done. Now, telemedicine and data transmission from an ICU would change this view, but I worry about not being able actually to touch the patient or to listen to the heart and lungs.

I cared for my mother's sister who was dying of terminal and painful adrenal metastatic cancer. I sat at her bedside through the night using the careful administration of morphine to blunt her pain. She died toward early morning. She looked, at times, so much like my own mother and I was especially glad to be there. At that time, the expectation was to care for dying patients at home. Family members were taught to give subcutaneous doses of morphine or Demerol dispensed in vials. These vials of narcotics were subsequently returned to the physician. I still do not understand the need for a Kevorkian when we have, at hand, effective opiates and other drugs that offer comfort and rest. We have forgotten how to give the attention that dying patients need, preferring, instead, to hide them away and to deny, at all costs, the inevitability of death.

Looking back, these were magical times in my medical career. The people I attended to and their loved ones understood death as an outcome. They were tough enough to recognize its inevitability. Today, we do save many more people with high-tech medicine, but clearly, people are not as happy with the care they receive now, as they were during those days of my first practice. I seem to recall rays of sunlight in those households.

It is said that we cannot go home again; yet, in my later practice, I returned again and again to those bright places and vivid lessons. A doctor doing house calls today could not survive in the Bronx or Mt. Vernon, where we had traveled and worked with impunity. Now, there would be danger of being mugged for the drugs in our black bags. Society and medicine have changed drastically. One would no longer dare treat acute pulmonary edema in the home. In that era, sophisticated monitoring, intensive care units and cardiac surgery did not exist. Our poor substitute was to sit at the bedside, observing hopefully for clinical improvement. Doing this led to a close rapport with patients and their families. And of course, this was inexpensive low-tech medicine. While good communication occurs in some of our units, I do not often see it. Families are excluded from the process of dying and cannot see how much we try to do for their loved one. Many times, we do too much, engendering unrealistic expectations and causing unnecessary discomfort at life's end. I hope to die at home.

During those months of general practice, many years ago, I learned medicine by observing sick people and their families. My bowling companions taught me unforgettable practical lessons in medicine and humanity. I also learned why medical work is called a *practice*. Whatever the medical circumstances, one seems to be rehearsing for the next case, always practicing. Though rarely used, I still keep the same black bag in my hall closet. I probably have accomplished much more in operating rooms under bright lights. But I still wonder about how best to serve. The magic of medicine still seems to reside in a black and mysterious bag. I continue to see medical problems as surprising and as novel as in those earlier days, and I see surgical challenges as exciting and as frightening now, as then. Practicing, whether as a specialist or a generalist, seems be of the same fabric. However simple or complex the illness, or the patterns of disease repeated, something novel always appears. Each lesson remains part of life and practice, to be recalled with great care. Each act, simple or complicated, is a rehearsal for the next.

LOOKING INTO PAST LIGHT

> It is as hard to see yourself as to look backward
> without turning around.
> Thoreau

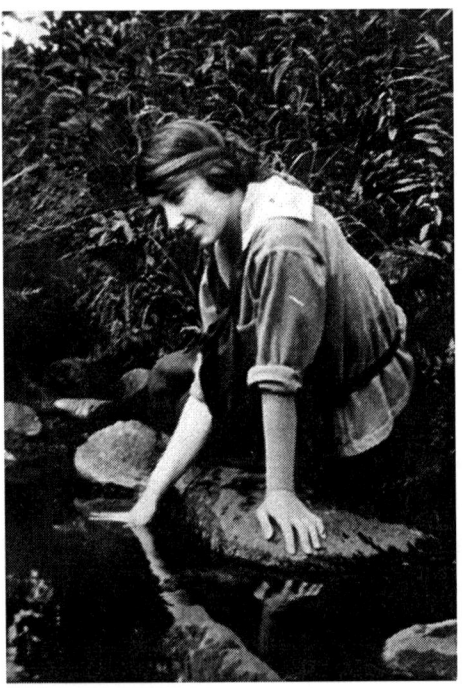

Maria Assunta Sibilio

Remembrances of childhood appear like motion pictures seen on an old-fashioned screen from the back row of a huge theater like Loews' Paradise on Fordham Road in the Bronx. Brightly illuminated scenes reappear. I see them under a violet sky with floating clouds and tiny stars in black and white, as movies were then; rarely, some images appear in color. Growing up Italian in the Bronx carried with it great advantages—large family gatherings, lavish Sunday dinners, and weddings with ice cream and cake—especially, it seemed, for children. Most of all, rays of sunlight seemed to shine upon children in those households. There was always something to look forward to. Events could mimic a Fellini film, complete with the scene in *8 and1/2* where a naked little boy is cuddled after bathing by ebullient aunts with great billowing breasts. These scenes appear to me now, just as they would in a movie, clearly though at some distance. With them comes a recognition that those women shaped our characters as men, making us, for better or worse, spoiled, confident in life, expecting much and receiving it from the women who loved us.

My first memory of home is a bright apartment on the top floor of a white six-story tower where we lived in the Bronx on Olinville Avenue, near Gun Hill Road. Our windows faced west, toward the park, with a view of the Bronx River bordered by weeping willow trees. A cat lived with us, too; we always had a cat. When *Alice in Wonderland* was first read to me, I visualized our cat as the Cheshire cat in the willow tree who would protect me from the Jabberwocky prowling the dense underbrush by the wall near the river. I came to have, in that place, two mothers. My mother, as the Depression was at its height, returned to school teaching when I was three, and Zaida Soldatini came from Milan to care for me. Zaida spoke "pure Italian" and my parents, ashamed of their Southern Italian dialects, hoped that I would learn proper speech from her. Exactly the opposite occurred. I was so terrified when Mother left me alone with Zaida for the first time, particularly since I could not speak with her, that I developed an antipathy—later regretted—to my parent's native language. Instead of my learning Italian, Zaida learned English. She was a large-boned, blue-eyed woman; loving and kind, and a single mother, which, in those times, presented many more problems than at present. Pregnancy, her embarrassment, had prompted her flight from northern Italy. I came to love her, in certain ways, more than my own mother. She stayed with us until I went to college, becoming the mainstay of our family life after my father died. She lived in fear of gypsies, who were known, or so she believed, to kidnap children in the old country. Much later, when I was ten years old, Dan Ryan, my best friend, and I dressed as gypsies, disguised in fake mustachios and earrings, and accosted her after sneaking into the kitchen through the cellar door of our house in Yonkers. She took one look at us and screamed, *"Auitame!"* and collapsed on the floor. Dan and I revived her, showing her our fakery in vain attempts at reassurance. She remained hysterical for hours. Our punishment was severe.

I spent the time of St. Genaro's feast at Zaida's downtown apartment in Little Italy. Later, when Zaida opened a boarding house in Long Beach, we spent several summer vacations on Long Island. There, as a young boy, my father taught me to swim in the rollicking Atlantic surf. Lunch was always something delicious—polenta, spinach and vegetables, and always ready when I came home from play or school. Zaida cooked dinners too—memorable pasta with beans, "pasta fazool," roasted chicken and potatoes and rice Milanese. She had a male companion, "Torridge," who had the demeanor of a large cat. He was a quiet, dark-eyed man with a gold tooth, a handlebar moustache framing a satisfied smile and either a toothpick or a small cigar protruding from the side of his mouth. He would drive us in a large sedan, usually a Packard or Buick, on the annual pilgrimage to Long Beach. Clearly, Torridge was a man to be reckoned with; he was probably "connected." During a bitter winter freeze, with fuel in short supply due to World War II, Torridge came with a dump truck to our home in Yonkers. After a serious conference with the owners of a coal yard, we carried precious "rice coal" on our backs to the truck for our bin. This was the only type of coal suitable for the stoker that heated our home. Torridge materialized whenever Zadia or our family needed something. We never asked questions and Torridge never offered explanations other than his gold-toothed smile. The Seven Santini Brothers took charge of our final move from New York to Cleveland in

1962, when my family relocated there as I completed surgical residency. The senior Santini himself gravely supervised the loading of furniture and the packaging of plates and glassware with great care. Every piece arrived in perfect condition in our new Cleveland Heights home. We understood this move ended an era; we had left New York forever.

My mother, Maria Assunta Sibilio, was a rebel, really an early feminist. She left her father's house against his wishes to attend teaching school and moved in with her sister, Genevieve De Felitta, who had married at age sixteen and lived near Fordham Road. Mother immigrated with her family from Monte Corvino Rovello, a small town north of Naples, to New York at the age of seven. She graduated valedictorian of her high school class ten years later. I read from her careful Palmer-style writing in a scrapbook how the family arrived in New York harbor in 1904, remaining on board overnight. We heard over and over how the lights of Manhattan appeared to be those of heaven, and indeed, for those southern Italians, they were. The name of her ship was *The Prince Albert*. At Ellis Island, an immigration officer spelled her family name wrong, "Sibera" rather than Sibilio. This mistake took years to correct. The new immigrants were too frightened or too diffident to argue with these imposing figures.

She had abandoned the Catholic Church after complaining about her father's tyrannies to a priest, who informed her that it was her confession, not her father's shortcomings, that needed discussion. She was outraged. Her father, my grandfather "Papanon," was a strong character who expected absolute obedience. As a result of her defection from Catholicism, during my early childhood, Mother attended various Protestant churches, a bewildering variety of them: Baptist, Methodist, and Episcopalian. These churches were, as she put it, clearly "American" and she wanted, above all, for us to be American. My father would have nothing to do with religion. To him, one "sky pilot" was like any other. These churches were scattered in the Bronx, Yonkers and Mt. Vernon. And, of course, I got to see them all.

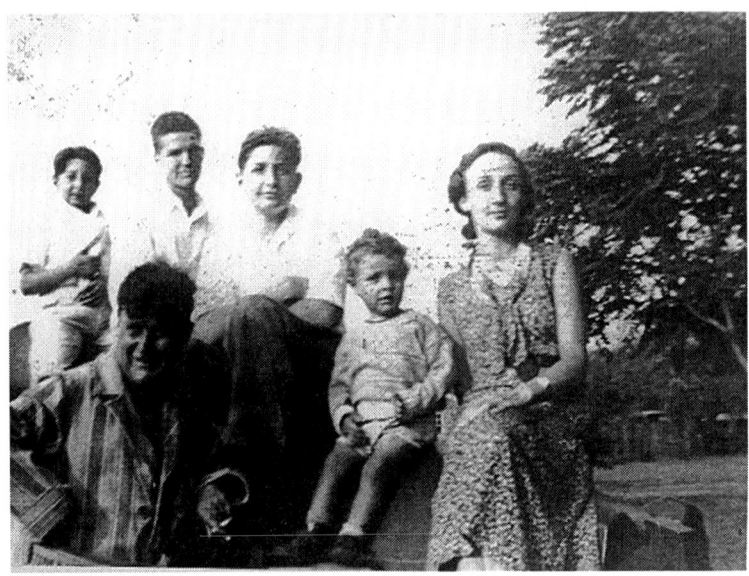

The Family: Left to right rear, Cousins Frank DeFelitta, Nicholas Sibilio, Buddy DeFelitta, and Grace DeFellita; Front Left, Frank DePalma, and author age two years. Staten Island, New York

The one I recall most vividly was a Baptist church, a large wooden structure with a high white steeple lurking in the shadow of the elevated on White Plains Avenue. There I became intrigued with their lurid depiction of leprosy, which the Baptists described in Sunday School. The images of fingers and toes falling off, blind people and facial disfigurements, were graphic and terrifying. After this indoctrination, I included in my nightly prayers "all people who are sick and with leprosy." I might have been rewarded for these specific prayers, for later, in medical school, we were given an unknown case in pathology as a problem in the form of autopsy slides. I recognized odd miliary granulomas—some involving nerves in what were clearly fingers—as leprosy. This unlikely and fortuitous diagnosis won me honors. Professor Von Glahn, an old school German pathologist, was initially incredulous and questioned me closely before awarding the honors grade. I told him of my childhood exposure to leprosy in the Baptist church, mentioning that slides of fingers and toes showing diseased nerves were critical clues for this diagnosis. The Old Prussian smiled tightly and held me in a quizzical gaze for a long time before dismissing me. He appeared pleased.

The problem with the various Protestant churches that mother attended was the prevalence of wacky scandals. Someone was always running away with someone else: the choir master with the minister's wife, the minister of yet another church with a choirgirl and on and on. So far as I knew, no one ran off with boys. The scandals invariably caused mother to become disenchanted. These experiences caused me to prefer Roman Catholicism where it seemed in those regal and authoritarian precincts, people behaved themselves, or at least, so it then appeared to my immature eyes. I had been baptized a Catholic at four, in the parish on Gun Hill Road. My father's sister, Aunt Albina, virtually abducted me to have this properly done. But not until I was fourteen was I confirmed as "Ralph Francis" and learned the proper Hail Mary and Act of Contrition. Mother later became a Christian Scientist when we lived in Cleveland. When she died, I had a mass said so she could be buried next to my father in the Gates of Heaven in Valhalla, New York.

After my father died in 1940, we were suddenly very poor. But Zaida stayed with us. She stood by our family through those terribly hard times. We paid her only forty dollars a month, but with that, she was able to raise a very fine daughter, Tina, who later worked at Macy's, in cosmetics. With a sense of glamorous adventure, we traveled downtown on the subway to Herald Square just to see Tina, tall and stately, presiding over her elegant domain. She later married an engineer and had a fine little boy who inherited my set of Lionel Standard Gauge Trains. I still think of those, the "big trains," as these are collectors' items now. I am glad, however, that this boy got this spectacular train set.

Father was a short, curly headed man. He was short-tempered, with piercing dark eyes, and was quick to remove his belt for any infraction or offense. He was generous, but if you asked or nagged for things, as children do, a negative outcome was certain. I learned

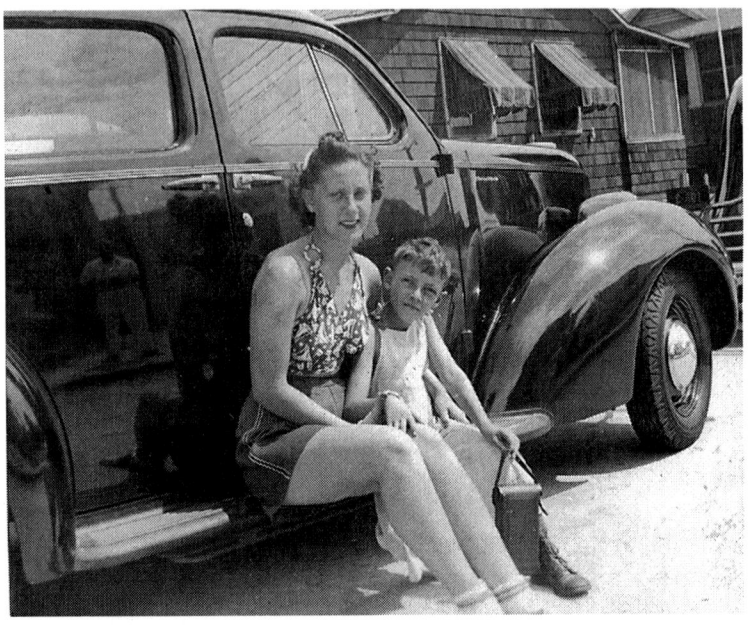

Tina Soldatini and the Author in Long Beach, Long Island, New York.

not to cross him and never, never to beg. He was, as my mother said, "God-fearing," though he never went to church. His trade was the fabrication of custom jewelry so favored by the ladies in the late 1930s. He and my Uncle Sam, a large, bald man, a tailor, co-owned a small shop on Maiden Lane where, in spite of the Depression, they had a thriving business in custom dresses and jewelry. Prosperity continued until Uncle Sam seduced the wife of an Irish police captain. My father was "God-fearing," according to mother, in that he did not, in contrast to his brother, chase women. Uncle Sam, on the other hand, liked what was in dresses even better than he liked dresses. So it came to pass that Samuel De Palma fled New York to Mexico, where he had remained, as World War II just started. We were at war with Italy by the time I was ten years old, and Uncle Sam was considered a hostile alien. From time to time, we received photographs of Sam surrounded by attractive ladies enjoying themselves at restaurants and floating barges. Mother and I would have to greet dark vivacious women arriving in New York styling themselves as *novias* or "wives" of Uncle Sam. These women were always exquisitely dressed and always stayed at the Algonquin Hotel to meet and entertain us. Then, after a decade, we heard no more from the Mexican ladies or about Uncle Sam.

Just before Sam and Frank DePalma parted company, my father, who stood five feet four inches, and his brother, had a monumental dispute in our living room. Arguments and recriminations raged in Italian and a bit of English as well. I crouched unobtrusively and listened from a corner of the room. My outraged father savagely berated Sam, standing a head taller, for his ramblings. By the end of this tirade, Sam cowered and looked truly contrite. In spite of his black sheep status, Sam, among thirteen uncles and aunts, will always be my favorite De Palma. When he visited, he never failed to bring a spectacular gift or substantial amount of money for those times, like a dime or a quarter. Once, he brought a real major league football. Scrutinizing old photographs, now that I am bald, I see that I resemble Uncle Sam, more than I do my father, Frank De Palma.

When I was six, we moved from Olinville Avenue to Hone Avenue, where we were closer to another branch of the De Palmas. Pre-World War II Sunday dinners were at Uncle Jimmy's and Aunt Albina's. During those bright days, the Yankees always won the ball games, Joe DiMaggio hit a home run, and the Bronx was the best place in the world. Smiling Jack and Dick Tracy of the comics in *The Daily News* won out over the bad guys, and all things were as they should be. Smiling Jack, the aviator, was our particular hero. Once, cornered by some really bad guys on a desert island, he escaped by building a glider out of his girlfriend's silk dress. Mortimer Sullivan, our landlady's son, took this feat seriously. He built a glider out of Mrs. Sullivan's best silk dress. Mounting a high billboard facing Boston Post Road, he prepared to launch himself from a height of sixty feet. Mortimer had waited until he could fly into a favorable northeast wind. We delayed him until his bewildered mother arrived to dissuade him from repeating Smiling Jack's feat. After we finally helped to get him down,

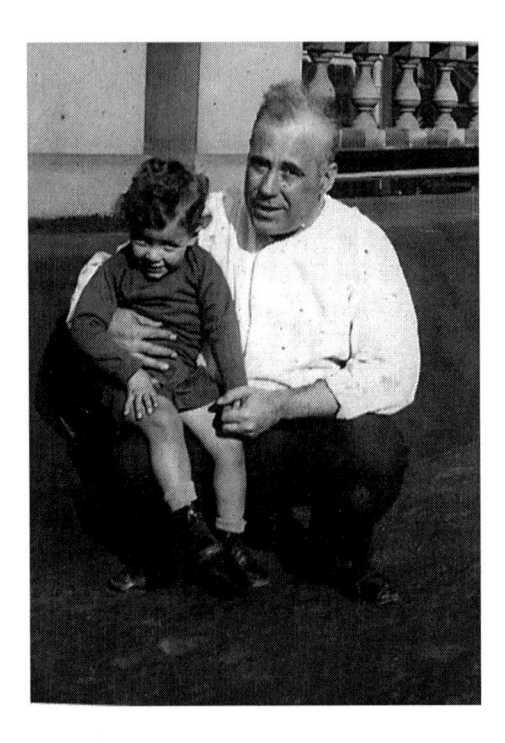

Uncle Samuel DePalma and the Author in Manhattan, New York

Mortimer was taken home in awesome silence, and we heard no more about his punishment, if any. While Mortimer was not exactly bright in any way, he was brave and certainly intrepid. I still wonder if the glider would have flown.

While the family argued over Mussolini at Sunday dinner, we could hear Hitler ranting ominously on the radio. The De Palmas were, by and large, violently antifascist. Some of them were even considered communists since they fought with The Lincoln Brigade in Spain. This might have caused difficulty, if it had been mentioned in my security clearance when I became an air force officer. In retrospect, I am proud of their politics during that era.

The family on that side also shared an anti-clericalist prejudice mainly among the men. Father was skeptical of organized religion, Social Security, and the draft. He predicted that Social Security numbers would be used to enslave us, an astute prediction. He said that the family left Italy to get away from these things—particularly from obligatory military service. His readings included *The Essays of Schopenhauer*, and *The Decline and Fall of the Roman Empire*. He and Gibbons attributed the unfortunate fall of Rome to the spread of Christianity. After reading these tomes myself, I understood why my father's perspective could be so negative

We went to the movies virtually every Saturday and Sunday. One day, when I was nine, my friend Nicky and I saw a newsreel at Lowe's Post Road, in which an Italian frogman swam into Gibraltar Harbor, placing a limpet mine, which successfully sank a British cruiser. The audience approved of their feat with wild applause. I ran home to our house on 216th Street with my friend Nicky Renzi to describe this triumph. Father's strap came off—I got a beating, and Nicky got a tongue-lashing. "Never forget that we came here because Italy gave us nothing." We were soon to be at war with Italy, and I guess he knew this with certainty.

However strict or gruff, father was also kind. We took long quiet walks—to the ballpark, to a lake in Bronx Park to sail a beautiful toy sailboat. He was acutely observant, and would point out things that most people might overlook. He finally had us move from 216th Street in the Bronx to Kimball Avenue in Yonkers, after my sister Grace was born. He and my mother bought a house and he died a year later. He wanted us to be upwardly mobile and saw no future in the old neighborhoods. Just before we moved, I became seriously ill, probably because of an incarcerated inguinal hernia, which was finally diagnosed by our general practitioner, Dr. Gerald Carroll. Mom and Dad borrowed $150 to pay the great Irish surgeon, Dr. Cunniff, of Union Hospital in the Bronx, to do the operation. My last recollection in the operating room, before smothering under the open ether mask, was Dr. Carroll's worried face hovering over me. I was confined to bed from May 10 till July 1 for recovery. I vomited for days and the wound, closed with clips, was crusted and painful for weeks. This was not the usual course of a childhood hernia repair today; nonetheless, after six decades, the repair remains quite solid.

Unfortunately, as a result of the imposed bed rest, I grew weak, and a move to an all-Irish neighborhood in Yonkers was an inopportune time to be weak. All the boys and even some of the girls in that neighborhood fought at least once a week; and from the age of ten until sixteen, one by one, I had to defeat each of my friends to obtain any peace at all. At thirteen, I secretly went to a gym on Riverdale Avenue to take boxing lessons from a feisty Golden Gloves coach who thought I might have promise. Having been converted from left to right-handedness, I remained relatively ambidextrous and my left jab and hook were strong. My adolescent growth spurt began early, and, at thirteen, I was five feet eight inches and one hundred and thirty pounds, soaking wet. My boxing career ended after a short black kid promptly closed my left eye then kept circling left, scoring numerous times. The coach thought I was getting cocky and wanted me to be challenged. He was right for I had seriously underestimated my small opponent. I heard birds and bells after the three obligatory rounds. Boxing, I decided, was unhealthy. I reasoned that, at some time and place, there would always be a superior adversary. But my boxing skills were honed enough to defeat all the neighborhood boys including Arthur, the toughest of all of them, who, after his decisive defeat, ran off to join the army when he was sixteen. I seldom picked fights and avoided confrontations.

But I did have a temper when provoked and I still, unfortunately, do. At four, a fat seven-year-old boy persistently harassed me while I was roller-skating on the concrete expanse in front of the Olinville School. He kept pushing me down from behind, taking my hat and being mercilessly abusive. Both my knees were bloody from repeated falls. It felt as if this pain would never end. I was wearing short pants, which left me unprotected from the coarse concrete sidewalk. I carefully secured my skate key from my jacket, unbuckled only one skate, and hopped up three steps leading to the school doors. This gave me necessary height and leverage, and I was able to strike him on the top of his head with an accurate downward blow. He collapsed, his nose copiously bleeding, unconscious, onto the pavement. He remained unconscious for a day. I was told later that his skull was fractured.

I felt neither triumph nor remorse. Zaida and the coterie of clucking Italian women were appalled. "Such a nice, quiet boy. How could he do this?" The seven-year-old was kept some distance from me after his long confinement.

Nothing was ever said to me about this incident and I was not punished. Looking back, the truth of the matter was, as Sowell has written in *Ethnic America* about Italians: "Casual brawling was to be avoided, but a serious fight was to be pursued implacably. In complete contrast to the Irish style of quick-to-anger and quick-to-forgive, the southern Italian pattern was one of polite but fair warning to head off trouble—and implacable vengeance if the other party persisted in offensive acts." Could it be that such characteristics, which I was certainly not taught, might be something genetic? Responsible adults need to settle scores by acceptable indirection, but I would prefer a direct approach in some instances. In discussing this failing of mine with a young Syrian whom I deeply respect, I pointed out that, in Islam, turning the other cheek is considered a sign of weakness. Anton, a Christian, replied, "Ralph, we read from another book." And he is probably right, but still, could there be a case for bringing back the custom of the duel? I believe that the fat bully would be unlikely repeat his behavior, at least, not without seriously weighing the consequences.

I never fought or even argued with Dan Ryan, my best boyhood friend. He was not given to brawling. He was a natural athlete and could accomplish any feat with his wiry, coordinated body. As young boys, we attended mass regularly on Sundays and during Lent on weekdays. I am sure that, had it not been for his early death, Dan would have become a priest. We had great times talking and joking, going to movies, church and boy scouting. I made Life Scout, but by fourteen, I became interested in girls, a serious distraction from the diligent pursuit of merit badges. Danny never showed this interest, nor did he exhibit the usual prurient adolescent preoccupations.

Abruptly, Dan began to spend all his spare earnings on Pepsi or Coke and Ho Ho cupcakes, insatiably gulping down sweets. At fourteen, he was hospitalized, requiring insulin for severe childhood diabetes, and he seemed to accept this illness with grace. We were close companions until I went to Roosevelt High School. Later, I only saw him during rare college breaks. He took me to drink beer at all-night bars, mostly in black neighborhoods. He was well liked and seemed to know all the regulars. But he was not supposed to drink at all, and he died at nineteen. Oddly enough, on the two occasions that I have been very ill, I have dreamed of seeing Dan, talking with him, and laughing at something or other, as he shared his quiet agreeable smile and wry humor.

My father's death was sudden. He became ill overnight after a brief period of intense itching, swollen legs and severe shortness of breath. I would now guess that his death was either cardiac or due to kidney failure. On the night that he died, I dreamed that we were taking our usual walk across a high and elaborate cantilevered bridge and, halfway across, he ordered me back. On my refusal, his hand moved toward his belt, "You cannot come," he seemed to say. The next morning, the family, gathered around in the kitchen, was afraid to talk to me. I reassured them that I knew Father had died. I had said my goodbye to him on that bridge.

Several comic episodes happened at my father's funeral. There was an open-casket viewing at the Boccino Funeral Home on Third Avenue, and the large family gathered, all sitting in rows. As four of my aunts stood contemplating his body, their ample and girdled behinds in black dresses were imposing, indeed. My cousin Georgie, then fourteen, looked at me sideways. I was crying a lot. He said, "Ralphie, look at that. There are twelve yards of ass." We have all been in situations where laughter seizes us inappropriately. This was one of those times; we could not stop laughing nor disguise our unseemly mirth. Georgie DePalma and I garnered dirty looks. At the interment in the Gates of Heaven Cemetery, one of the aunts, my father's younger sister, jumped down on the coffin as it was being lowered into the ground. This gesture was an astonishing and shocking event for me, since my mother's family was not at all demonstrative. They hoisted her out with great effort, spilling half of a large breast and elaborately gartered thighs from her straining black dress. But in spite of the violent mourning gestures, Mother got little help from her husband's family. We rarely saw the De Palmas again. Why this was so escapes me. It might have had something to do with my mother and her religious beliefs, though she denied that. I was told some of them owed us money.

Father's death left Mother in severe financial straights. Because of his skepticism about insurance and Social Security, Father never purchased insurance nor would he even obtain a Social Security number. He was strongly opinionated, and while logic was on his side, he was clearly wrong. We had only Mother's earnings from teaching to support my sister and me, along with debts and the mortgage on the house. She always worried, poor Mother, about money, and her feet hurt. After a lifetime of standing in operating rooms, my feet now hurt, so I know how she must have felt. I have seen to it that my family was adequately insured. When Mother could no longer live with us, she went to the Amasa Stone Nursing Home in Cleveland. At eighty, her Alzheimer's became dangerously disabling. She would get on a Cleveland Heights bus and ask the driver to take her to 238th Street and White Plains Road to get to her school on Lenox Avenue and 135th Street in Harlem, where she had taught for thirty-five years. The patient bus drivers, mostly African American, would gently return her to our house, a large municipal bus nosing up our driveway. She would alight, cheerfully thanking the smiling driver. Her wandering and serious falls, one of which caused a hip fracture, mandated her admission to a nursing home. My wife had been generous in sharing our household with her, as I was later glad to have Eve's mother, Grace Tankard, living with us in McLean, Virginia.

Mother always appeared to be sweet and diffident, and these characteristics seemed magnified by her senile delusions. On the other hand, at times, she could become implacably stubborn. After the agitation began, she once insisted that there was a mistake in the sums of her bank accounts. On investigation, she was correct; the bank had made an error of $50. When I was driving her to the nursing home, she turned, looked at me and said, "Don't look so glum. You lived with me for seventeen years, and I lived with you for seventeen years." She died of pneumonia at eighty-six. I had taken her financial account and invested it conservatively during the high interest rates occasioned by the Carter years. Try as I might to reassure her that she would not run out of money, she remained fearful of this her whole life. In the month that she died, in spite of careful husbanding of her pension and the proceeds from the sale of the Yonkers house, exactly $249 remained. Mother had two funerals: one Protestant, in Cleveland, attended by her many loyal African American lady friends, and one in Westchester, for the Catholic contingent. After my father died, because my mother had no money, she had not ordered a stone to mark the site of the grave. She was almost buried in the wrong plot when my daughter, Malinda, recognized her great grandmother's name, Philomina, on a nearby gravestone. By speaking up, her granddaughter prevented the same serious error as had occurred on my mother's entry to this country. The cemetery staff quickly corrected the error, and a new grave was opened in the proper site. I bought a large monument and saw to it that it was placed at the head of the De Palma plot.

On a trip of remembrance, I hired a car and drove from the Plaza Hotel to all those old places in the Bronx. The resplendent tower on Olinville Avenue looked so small and shabby now. The houses on Hone and 216th Street appeared about the same size as I remembered them. The Bronx inhabitants were now good-natured Hispanics. At Olinville Avenue, they were kind enough to let me look around, and a cheerful Puerto Rican family invited me into our old apartment on the sixth floor. In spite of humble furnishings and a faint foreign cooking odor, it seemed to me that the bright light was still shining in that place. I looked at the school steps and the broad expanse of concrete where I used to roller skate. The Kimball Avenue house in Yonkers still had an Italian stone wall my father and my uncle, Pat DeFelitta, built by hand half a century before. The stones were carefully fitted; no mortar had been used. They both died soon after all their strenuous labor finishing that home.

I did not go in.

How brave they were—all of them—in searching for a better life for us. A bluff stone monument marks the plot at the Gate of Heaven. Looking back in time, I see bright lights and fires on a screen that shaped our lives. I have fond remembrances of my Bronx childhood, a motion picture playing forever in my mind's eye. On a recent trip to Buenos Aires, I saw these words written on a wall in the neighborhood they call Boca, The Mouth, where it faces the harbor, "*Ya vienen los immigrantes y las estrellas cayen desde el cielo.*" The immigrants came and the stars fell from the heavens. In New York, half a hemisphere away, when my family came as immigrants, I believe stars also fell from heaven.

RAT RACES

Infirmity alone makes us take notice and learn.
Proust

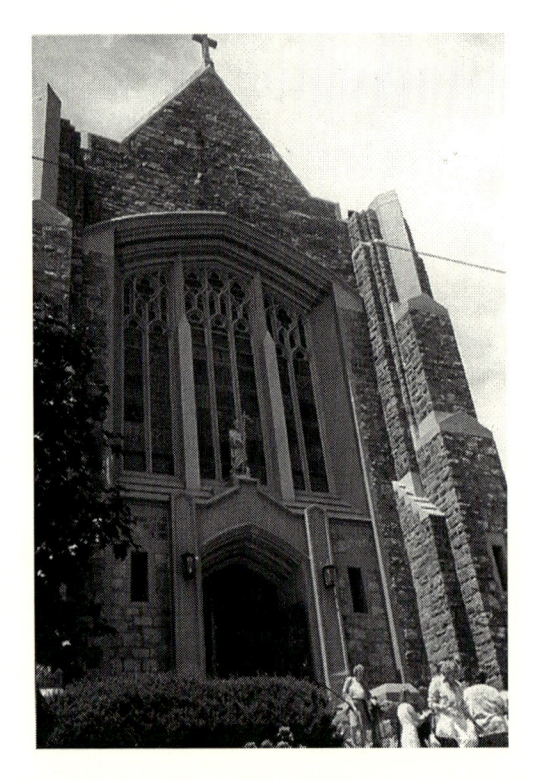

Saint John the Baptist Church, Yonkers, New York

    For a long time, I used to stay in bed late. Sometimes, I would open my eyes when it got light, but when I turned on my side, my eyes would close so quickly the conscious thought that "I am going to sleep again" never surfaced. Simply agreeable sensations and soft pillows and sweet dreams seemed to have currents of their own, and, half an hour later, I thought I should awaken, but I could never ask myself the time. Instead, on mornings when I slept late, time was punctuated by a sequence of exquisite cooking odors. On Saturdays, the odor of bacon and pancakes, and on Sundays, the unique spicy smell of homemade gravy for pasta, awakened my senses. On holidays, there might be the odor of pizza on Easter morning, or, on Christmas, zeppola, a kind of deep-fried doughnut soaked in honey. I loved sleeping late and now, I wish I still could. But a call roused me from childish reveries. The Rat Races began.

We lived, at the time, in Yonkers, an ethnic suburb, north of New York City. Its main street bordered the eastern shore of the Hudson River. The hilly town was studded by neighborhoods—each with its own parish, each on top of a hill, and each delineated a neighborhood, and each, in fact, a cultural microcosm. The spires of these hilltop churches aimed at the very heart of heaven. The churches were named for the company of saints: St. Joseph, St. John, St. Catherine, and so on. Some of the parishes were predominately Polish, such as the one on Nodine Hill. Our parish, St. John's, was mixed Irish and Italian, but the Irish predominated in both congregation and the clergy. Teenagers congregated at various social clubs such as the Catholic Youth Center, the YWCA, and the YMCA, where Tuesday nights through Sunday nights, we danced to records at one or another of church basements or institutional halls. On weekends, live music ruled at the Polish Community Center on Nodine Hill, with spectacular Polka bands, kielbasa, and generous jugs of beer for those of us who looked old enough. Boys and girls could meet at these affairs, pair off, dance, and then date. Boys were looking for random sexual adventures, but by age sixteen, young women at these dances were mostly playing for keeps, looking for marriage. High-collared priests at the Irish Catholic parishes kept a careful eye on the dancers, using a stick or a knurled cane to separate couples who became too entwined during slow dancing. The churchmen had a two-fold conflicting goal: they needed marriages and offspring for new parishioners, but they required a courting ritual, even as they strove to keep the swirling couples from serious occasions of sin. These dances, in humble and slightly tawdry halls, substituted for the debutante balls of Manhattan, but on a much larger and effective scale, as they occurred so often at one parish or another in the hilly city. The fact that we went virtually every night of the week from one place to another, to pair off and dance, led to naming these frenetic affairs "Rat Races." As much biological as social functions, boy-girl couplings at the dances became tantalizing exercises in temptation and restraint. Unlike the debutante circuit, no dancing school prepared us, but during that time, we somehow became excellent ballroom dancers.

Sometimes we went downtown to Manhattan, to Roseland, a glamorous ballroom on Broadway where we danced to live music, usually two bands: one Latino and one American. At Roseland, by an unwritten rule, the better dancers got to perform closer to the bandstand. My regular dancing partner was a tiny sweet girl named Connie from a slum in Yonkers near Riverdale Avenue. She had sparkling blue eyes and chestnut hair, which she wore neatly coifed about her face like a helmet. At about 4 feet 10 inches, she weighed 95 pounds, making her easy to lift for the acrobatics demanded by the lindy hop. She followed any subtle lead in the tango or complicated close-couple dances like the peabody or fast two-step. Connie and I concentrated on dancing. We rarely talked about anything at all. Not that talking mattered much, for in these close fast-moving dances, it was impossible to chat. Most serious dancing required absolute concentration, as many of the moves were executed without forethought and the woman had to respond to subtle clues from her male partner. Undoubtedly, we appeared to be a sophisticated couple, but we were really naïve seventeen-year-old kids who simply just liked to dance.

The next year, I went to Columbia College. At the request of my second semester English teacher for an essay about a girlfriend, I wrote about Connie, and our dancing adventures, particularly, advancing to the front of Roseland. The professor, a chubby sarcastic man who styled himself an "Austenian scholar," also wrote sardonic reviews for the *New York Times*. I was shocked to receive a C for this essay. I had gotten straight A's in writing in the prior semester. He invited me to discuss the essay in his dingy cluttered office. Finally, he got to the point, asking with a fat-faced smirk, "Did Connie screw?" My omission of the details of this aspect of our relationship was clearly the reason for the C. Appalled by his demeanor and crudeness, I gave no answer and left. I was determined to apply myself to science, where, so I believed at the time, performance could be assessed more objectively. Apparently, some adults in the upper echelons of the Columbia College faculty did not share the fastidious sense of honor current among seventeen-year-old lower-class Bronx boys. This nosy fellow went on to become headmaster at a waspy boy's prep school. I guess the parents of those boys got their money's worth. Not that we didn't fool around, but we rarely discussed this publicly. Even so, we had to face confession once a month on Saturday night. "Are you married? Is she married?" the priest asked, following whatever answer by stern admonitions.

At St. John's, the senior pastor, Father Barry, grumbled just loud enough in the confessional so that all in the waiting line might catch a key word or two. Father Barry, an Irishman of strong opinions, believed in Monsignor Sheehan and William Randolph Hearst. The editorial policies of *The Journal American* approached in his mind the catechismal truth. For any sin of the heart, the penitent had to do prayers at each of the Stations of the Cross, indicating to the parishioners a probable carnal sin of some sort. We had learned that the Kimball Avenue bus, easily and discretely, reached the Italian church at a place called Nanny Goat Hill, named after the immigrants who raised goats there. Whenever sins of the heart were to be confessed, we visited this particular church, a humble squat Romanesque structure. Many of the priests there did not speak English well; those that did were serious and sympathetic. Penance routinely consisted of five or ten Our Fathers and Hail Mary's and an Act of Contrition. We could then attend communion the next day, facing the glorious gothic apse at St. John's where Father Barry would eye us suspiciously. He was keeping track. However, at the Italian church, a single mention of doubts about our faith or of criticism of our parents caused severe repercussions, including post-confessional conferences. This was fitting, as I came to see later. Dante had the illicit lovers, Paulo and Francesca, entwined with each other in eternal embrace, blown about by hot winds on the outskirts of Hell. In contrast, heretics, liars and hypocrites were frozen alive in ice in the depths of the inferno. These sinners, in the Italian scheme, were considered unforgivable. Some speculate about Catholic guilt, but infusions of guilt did little permanent harm and I suspect that liberal attitudes somehow later affected even some priests. The fire and ice of romantic attraction and sinful danger even made relationships between boys and girls more thrilling. At the least, we learned to take sex—heterosexual sex—for the high but dangerous adventure it could be. We knew no one who might be gay.

At Roosevelt High School, a magnet academic school, I began to lose touch with my childhood neighborhood friends. Some students came from the old Yonkers neighborhoods, and others, a more upscale part of Westchester County. Roosevelt High, dominated by principal Henry "Hank" Richards, stressed the philosophy that all students were pointed towards college. This was fortunate, for it took me a while to get this idea, though without having to study, academic success and high grades seemed to come easily. I began to take athletics seriously, too. Long summers surfing as a child in the Atlantic paid off. I became a serious swimmer. During my junior and senior years, I held city and county records for backstroke. Mr. Richards, a grizzled burly man, was a stern disciplinarian. Miscreants were grabbed by the nape of the neck and bodily transported to his office. We lived in fear of him and this was totally appropriate.

Apart from books, which I read unceasingly, my first inkling that a life of the mind existed was exposure to plane geometry and sublime satisfaction derived from writing *quat et demonstratum* or *reductio ad absurdum* at the end of the proof. It was thrilling to know something with that kind of certainty. The challenge of a Scottish mathematics teacher led me to solve the cosine theorem without reference to a book. I did this one bright afternoon in the beginning of my junior year, thus developing a serious affinity for mathematics and physics. The appearances of symbols and equations on paper were beguiling. They described an almost otherworldly but real place, and at the same time, real truths for the real world. As denominators approached zero, the value of fractions spiraled into real but universal infinity. After a competitive examination, where I performed best in mathematics, I was chosen to work in the physics research laboratory of Alexander Smith and Sons, a carpet factory in the Saw Mill River Valley.

Here, a reserved and curiously sad former atomic scientist taught me calculus to measure high polymer fiber behavior under bending and stretching stress. We published "The Bending Modulus of Single Wool and Synthetic Fibers" in a technical journal. I fully intended a career in physics, but there were many other things I needed to do which did not, in the least, interest my peers in the laboratory. There were the Rat Races, and daily swimming practice during summer and winter. My two best friends at the time were not aspiring physicists but a Polish kid from Nodine Hill, Drew, and a flamboyant Italian, Ernie, from Riverdale Avenue. Uncharitably, it could be said that they were blue-collar, but they were loyal and affectionate friends and much more fun than young scientists. We sang as a trio and one of our dreams was to join the navy, save money and open a bar where we would sing. Our trio actually performed in little bars and we got food and drinks for these efforts. When we were sixteen, we tried to enlist in the navy. This might have happened but the recruiting officer spotted the fact that my friends and I were under age. In addition, I failed the Ishihara Color Blindness Test. Not to be defeated in all of this, we then joined the famous Seventh Regiment of the New York National Guard, satisfying a thirst for military glory in time for the Korean conflict. Luckily, the war ended and we did not have to serve overseas. But one of our friends from the Yonkers Regiment died at Yalu.

The nightly Rat Races continued, and the girls we met at them, from Polish, Hungarian, Irish, and Italian parishes, entered and left our lives in a never-ending colorful swirl. I managed to buy, for $120, a 1933 Plymouth Coup with a rumble seat for transport as well as for the other social essentials. I started driving at fifteen with a learner's permit, which was illegal after sunset. This did not deter any us from primetime nocturnal driving. One of the first things I did was take a date, a sweet blond named Effie, to an ill-advised parking spot near Sprain Lake Golf Course. Fortunately, before anything much happened, big flashlights, blue suits and badges gleamed in the steamed-up windows. We were ordered to step out. One of the officers said to his partner: "Arrah d'ya see who this girl is?" I didn't know, but soon found out. She was the daughter of their police lieutenant. After severe reprimands, they sent us home contrite and relieved. Luckily, I did not lose my privileges to drive, as this action on their part, they told me, would have alerted Effie's father, and surely, "He would have killed us both." Besides, Rat Races were in full progress; I needed the car.

In the spring of my senior year, an attractive lady, our English teacher, assigned us a Eugene O'Neil play, a morbid family thing of his depressing genre. She asked me publicly what I would do in case of such a dysfunctional entrapment. I said, "Well, simply leave—walk out." She was visibly shocked by this terse answer. Agitated, she suddenly screeched out: "Haven't you ever been in love?" Her response was so emotionally exaggerated that I could not, for a moment, reply. The whole class was staring. Her response to my ill-considered answer had touched some painful inner spot. I thought to myself, "Maybe I have, but not enough to suffer all this." She listened attentively as I described my busy schedule, explaining that this would not leave time for O'Neil's maundering. She replied, again with emotion, "Ralph, you are too busy doing too much," an exasperated female message I was to hear over and over. A couple of girls wrote in my yearbook to ask if I had yet been in love. I figured there was time for that later. There were races to run. I was having too much fun to stop, to think too much or to get caught in a biologic mantrap, no matter how attractive the bait. At certain times, thinking too much is a bad thing. These thoughts are philosophic heresy, the unexamined life and all that. But the time for introspection was not during races. To quote Yogi, "You can't think and hit."

But now I look back to the shining faces of old friends and feel the spirit of that time, in that town, with high-slated church steeples. I might have been a better teacher, had it not been for a streak of severity in judging others, a peculiar impatience with myself, and a desire for prompt actions on the part of others. David Smith, my swimming coach and director of the Yonkers YMCA, encouraged my swimming career. He was a bald, vivacious man who lined me up to swim against the freshman team at Columbia, which earned me a scholarship when I beat both of their freshmen as well as their varsity backstrokers. I recall the intense interest and the demands of the fine faculty at Roosevelt High School.

Fifty years later, at a class reunion, I realized that Michael and David Halverstam were alumni. But I had not known them or thought to seek to know them. The class of 1949 displayed a generous sprinkling of professional men, a dean, an Admiral of the Navy, various doctors, lawyers, and smooth ad agency people. After fifty years, the curious amalgam of blue collar and upper class remained. I still feel the generosity and sensitive warmth of the sad physicist at the carpet factory and the affections of my teenage companions, now long gone. Some did not want me to leave them. When I began to get my name in the paper for swimming, friends in the old neighborhood, save for Dan Ryan, resented the publicity, saying that I was "showing off." It was a long time before I could consciously seek recognition. My old friends did not approve, but other, newer friends, did. During that time and place, I was roused from sleeping late in Yonkers to join the races. Those races and their urgencies now seem diminished, but I am yet eager to compete in some way. During a recent serious illness, I searched for the meaning of those lost times and recalled their sweetness.

Perhaps a few of my old friends had been right. It might have been better to remain anonymous in the old neighborhood and to settle there. This was our Combray on the Hudson. Perhaps, the concerned English teacher was right. Doing things, rather than feeling things, might not be the best way of life. Perhaps, Father Barry was right. He believed that we should count on God only and not look to other human beings for happiness. More questions now come, rather than answers. Yet, even now, I am still torn between races and reveries. But I now embrace journeys into a languorous past and its sweet late-morning dreams. Searching back, I fall into a deep slumber, sometimes visited by a mysterious asthenic spirit, not knowing whether my eyes will open or whether I shall be able to take my next breath. Yet, I am neither afraid nor unhappy. It is as if I now live in those remembrances and, at the same time, exist on the cusp of something quite new.

THE LION THAT BARKED

> For a man to achieve all that is demanded of him he must regard himself as greater than he is.
> Goethe

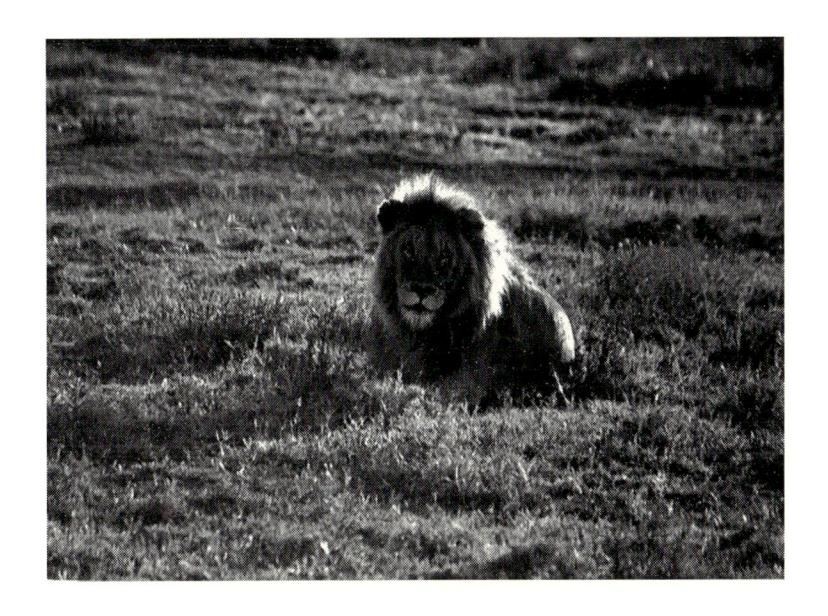

Lion in the Seringeti, 1996

Lions do not commonly roar. On a Safari, we slept one night in tents on the Serengeti, near a pride of lions gathered a few hundred yards from our camp. Our guides placed lanterns front and back and warned us not to walk outside that night. In our tents, we heard a series of low-pitched barks and woofs in descending crescendos, which, the guides told us, were the male lions speaking Swahili. Their bark was to let other animals know that they were lions and that they were kings. The deep sounds were benign but authoritative. That night, we slept restlessly but the lions did not bother our camp. Noisy, marauding hyenas did. The anthem "Roar Lion Roar" woke no echoes at all in the Hudson Valley at Columbia College in 1949. The Columbia Lions won few football games, but did better at basketball and baseball mainly because of athletes from campus fraternities. The Roar Lion hymn seemed pretentious.

While Columbia was intellectually unchallenged, its football team was mediocre. Just after I went to Columbia College, Dwight D. Eisenhower became the university president, and his influence was to have a profound influence upon my education. Eisenhower appeared, from time to time, as a guest instructor for our contemporary civilization course, where we read from detailed and original sources. Discussions of the readings were intense, opinionated and contentious. The class had a proportion of New York commuters, many, leftist in their leanings. Eisenhower, a quiet and reserved man from Kansas, appeared to be quite moderate and possibly respectful of our exaggerated and dramatic opinions. He responded remarkably to our section when we condemned atomic warfare. We had been considering Bertrand Russell's recent essays that recommended a complete ban on atomic weapons. General Eisenhower then said that Russell had recently changed his mind on that issue. The statement seemed unbelievable. With his infectious smile and diffident manner, Eisenhower replied, "Well, Lord Russell is a friend of mine, maybe I can get him to come to discuss his views."

Two months later, Lord Russell came from England to speak at the Macmillan Theater on Broadway and 116th Street. To our astonishment, he recommended that we use atomic bombs against the Soviet Union in a first strike! Our jejune classroom challenge and Eisenhower's quiet response gave us a sobering glimpse of reality in world affairs. Russell's was an irresponsible and scary prescription, and Eisenhower publicly, and quite pleasantly, disagreed with him on stage that night. Eisenhower also made two remarks in passing that remained with me over the years. One was that, no matter who his boss was, he tried always to do the best job possible, whether he liked him or not. He was likely referring to General

McArthur. The second, and more relevant, was his wry statement that going bald never hurt his social life. I began to lose my hair as an undergraduate. This was comforting and also true. I became an Eisenhower Republican.

My scholarship, partly for swimming, was supplemented by a New York Regents Scholarship. But Columbia's swimming pool was out of commission during my freshman year and I did poorly. The team shuffled off to dismally crowded municipal pools, which were not really suitable for competition. Subway travel in midwinter made our swimming practice disorganized and sporadic. My first choice for colleges had been Rutgers, which had a fine Olympic-sized pool. Rutgers had an intensely organized athletic program and had also offered an academic scholarship covering tuition, but not living expenses. Since even living expenses were too much for Mother's limited resources, Columbia was a second choice. The money I had managed to save during summer work, as a lifeguard, was sufficient if I lived at home. Going to Columbia was a matter of lucky chance, not of deliberation. I began my studies with a major in physics and mathematics. Rutgers had offered a fascinating mathematical program involving actuarial predictions. Columbia gave me a scholarship of $400 annually, which was then reduced to $200 after I had won a $400 New York Regents' scholarship based upon a competitive examination which included mathematics, English composition, and, oddly enough, interior decorating. Studying interior decorating before the examination boosted my score enough for me to qualify. The combined sums of the scholarships, $600, came a bit short of tuition costs.

My brief interview at Columbia was low key and even casual, compared to the two-day grilling at Rutgers. When asked to describe my current readings, I gave an over-enthusiastic impression of the essays of Thomas Huxley. The interviewer gently deprecated my enthusiastic opinion of Huxley's simple rationalism. I suppose he was surprised to see a denizen of the Bronx contemplating any philosopher at all. After this interview, I was told that I was accepted. Only much later did I realize my good fortune. As fall began, I had little time to see my old friends in Yonkers. As a day student,

I commuted from Yonkers in what was called the "pastrami brigade." Between classes, the polyglot commuters from the various boroughs of New York congregated in John Jay Hall to study and wolf down sandwich lunches while studying.

The great courses at Columbia, humanities and contemporary civilization, required massive amounts of reading and thought. Beginning with the Greek philosophers and playwrights, we moved through Rabelais and the essays of Montaigne and Voltaire. My encounter with the Anthon Professor of Greek and Latin, Gilbert Highet, yielded an unforgettable first impression. On the first day, he literally bounded into the classroom at Hamilton Hall. Hearing Highet's English accent, I thought that he might be effete. Accents such as this were not heard in the Bronx. He also pulled a handkerchief out of a French-cuffed sleeve during his first lecture. He proved, however, to be a happily married Episcopalian. His wife was Helen McInnis, the mystery novelist.

His lectures and our class discussions fascinated me but I found his accent hard to follow. He also commented on my speech, the usual nasal New York horror that, up until then, had seemed normal to me. I was sent to remedial speech therapy. This I thought rather insulting. I was obliged to sit for hours listening to my own recitations on a creaky Dictaphone and comparing my own speech to proper accents. The drill was relentless. By the time I moved to the Midwest, the New York accent had changed into the flat tones of that part of the country. Under stress, however, the New York whine reappeared from time to time and I had to remain on guard to avoid this. This regional speech pattern, with its underlying attitude, might be responsible for the apparent irritability of New Yorkers. Highet, aware that he was dealing with the equivalent of a cockney accent, concluded that I needed help badly.

Polycarp Kusch, later to win a Nobel Prize in cryophysics, taught freshman physics. For chemistry, we used Linus Pauling's beautifully illustrated new book demonstrating chemical valences based on orbital electron exchanges. My first year thus became an exciting intellectual adventure. Solid geometry and calculus did not require much effort for me. So, for the first months, I stayed at home, commuting from Yonkers and continuing to enjoy home cooking and motherly attentions. At midterms, I found myself on the dean's list. The voluminous readings in the humanities and contemporary civilization were time-consuming but pleasurable. Highet's lectures in the humanities were something I looked forward to every day, and even his weekly quizzes were fun.

My studies, by subtle degrees, were gradually transforming my attitudes and beliefs. I became more skeptical of religion after reading Thomas Aquinas and considering "natural law," which did not seem natural at all to me. The bawdy good humor and sex in Rabelais' writings made the life of the body funny as well as fun and not at all shameful. Just before Christmas, we read Lucretius' *On the Nature of Things*. I, then, concluded that religion was probably largely nonsense. I had just turned eighteen and, for the first time, became terribly lonely. I missed my old friends who sinned with aplomb, confessed and then, attended mass. I had little time to spend with them and, even when we met for a beer, we seemed to have little in common to talk about. My new life was so distant from the old neighborhood. The physics and mathematics majors were uninteresting and what young people today call "nerdy." Worse, to my old friends, I, myself, had become a nerd. Though I was close to Yonkers, I felt lost.

And so, Christmas vacation of my first year was traumatic. I did not go to mass; I had become an atheist, or, at least, an agnostic. Highet, a devout Episcopalian, had taught three proofs of God's existence: 1) the need for a prime mover, 2) the apparent existence of order in nature, 3) the fact that, everywhere and in every place, men believed in the existence of a deity. I could not reconcile secular philosophy with a specific belief in the personal God that my faith taught. It seemed vain to think that God would have personal preferences in the infinite scheme of the cosmos. How did He keep track? A big, divine computer can easily solve this objection, but the concept of such powerful intelligence appeared beyond comprehension at the time. It seemed probable that things happened for no reason at all. Quite suddenly, I was looking at the void and the void looked back. A recent Columbia graduate, Leon Dominic Marrano, called me at home in Yonkers. He invited me to pledge with Beta Theta Pi, an old and respected fraternity founded in 1849 in Oxford Ohio. The chapter house at West 114th Street, an old five-story brownstone, ultimately became my home. After several months of hazing followed by "hell week," I became a brother in the Alpha Alpha chapter in the spring of 1950. This was a real turning point in my life. The chapter roster consisted of a preponderance of Anglo-Saxon names. I had joined a new kind of tribe. These new friends took me further and further from my old life and friends. I still dated girls from the old neighborhood, like Joni Pasquale and Trish O'Riley. The brothers treated these young women with great courtesy, but these girls were never comfortable at fraternity parties. They never seemed to fit in. Leon had been one of the first Italians in the fraternity; then there were others. The president one year was Ernie Petruleo. Eric Moses Javitts became the first Jewish brother and later became president. He was hazed unmercifully and was required to wear a yarmulke while he was a pledge. He did this with good grace and dignity.

Two senior veterans, fighter pilots, initially dominated the chapter. One of them, Charles Burgie, was interested in the progress of the new brothers. He was a master of mischief as well. We had to paint the walls of the party room burgundy; Burgie believed in Skinnerian behavioral psychology. All behaviors, human or animal, could be explained by positive or negative conditioned reflexes. He believed in sports and was a varsity javelin thrower. In his opinion, hot dogs, football, apple pie and anticommunism were the strengths of the country. He was Swiss and disliked Catholicism. "The Pope was digging a tunnel to the White House." He later became a stockbroker advising me to buy IBM stocks in 1957. His prescient advice helped my wife and me to purchase our first home many years later.

The fraternity activities on weekends featured a cast of characters presaging *Animal House*. A chubby Swedish brother from Minnesota engineered midwinter "glug parties". Glug was a kind of eggnog—thick, sweet, and intoxicating. We had a "barf hole" in the wall reputedly to be used after drinking excess glug. "Purple Jesus," a mixture of gin, vodka, grape juice and dry ice, smoked and bubbled in a large bowl at most parties. This concoction tasted completely benign but was exceedingly intoxicating. The hope was that girls would drink enough to abandon their inhibitions. However, female abandon was uncommon among college girls in the 'fifties. We were not supposed to take girls above the second floor, but we did. This environment was safer than the back seat of a car or a New York Park bench. None of us ever used drugs other than alcohol and cigarettes. We were discreet to the point of hypocrisy. While we had "toga parties" with no underwear, we also sponsored a solemn black tie formal at Christmas with girls who were courted seriously.

We chanted dreadful songs and limericks, which I learned to accompany, plucking on a tenor ukulele:

> *In days of old there lived a maid, who used to ply a roaring trade, it was a trade of ill repute, and in fact she was a prostitute.*
>
> *There also lived a giant tall, who with his cock could smash a wall, who daily fornicated all the harlots of Jerusalem.*

This went on, chorus after raucous chorus, describing the copulative encounter in Rabelaisian detail. There was an ode to Lydia Pinkham, and her love for the human race:

> *She made, she made her vegetable compound, and all the papers published her face.*

We celebrated Princess Papaya of Hawaii:

> *How'ja like to have a little bit of the Princess Papaya's papuya, they say she's giving it away.*

We held generic open houses on Friday nights: one night for nurses, one night for stewardesses, one night for Barnard girls. This was arranged so that the female underground, a powerful network, could not keep track of our dating patterns. Saturday night was reserved for serious dates. Eventually, I changed my pattern of dating Bronx girls when one of them, a beautiful hairdresser, passed out and vomited en route to an otherwise promising upstairs sortie. Clearly, we were being initiated, after a fashion, into a primitive form of social life. We were a close approximation, if not the exact sort of men Sylvia Plath described, but none of the women I knew reacted quite with as much anguish as she. Strict rules applied. Our limited weekend interactions were less stressful than those in the later coed dormitories where constant sexual tension was inescapable. Another thing about college in those times was that much more sexual activity occurred amongst middle-class Bronx kids than there was to be found in the college crowd—bravado, songs and Purple Jesus notwithstanding. I used to date a girl from the south Bronx and once, as we were taking a moonlit walk by the East River, I started to recite a bit of poetry. She turned to me saying, "Shut up and fuck me." Women from those precincts knew what they wanted.

In fraternity life, we were expected to be serious and respectful toward special long-term relationships with women. The seniors set the example. The Beta pin contained a tiny diamond, *"gem of gem that ne'er grows dim,"* and was considered as an engagement pledge. This was my first gift to my future wife. It was the only real jewelry I could afford at that time. A proper engagement ring waited until after my discharge from the military service, when we finally had money. Elizabeth Taylor, so beautiful after *National Velvet*, attended some of our parties as the date of a wealthy brother. He eventually gave the prized Beta pin to Elizabeth and, at the same time, to three other women. The chapter expelled him after a tumultuous meeting. Elizabeth went on to collect many bigger and better diamonds. One of the varsity wrestlers took to jumping apelike onto tables to announce that he was going to drop his drawers, which he then did. The first time or two, it was funny, but with repetition, these antics became offensive. An official censure duly recorded in the chapter minutes devastated him. He pled to have these minutes expunged, but this censure remains, as far as I know, in the permanent minutes of Alpha Alpha chapter. There were limits. The morality of the 'fifties prevailed. On several occasions, we wired the ladies' bathroom. The overheard remarks transmitted were startling, enlightening, but mostly, deflating and we never did this again.

Some men could never get dates. A now wealthy banking magnet focused on local girls he picked up at neighborhood dances at John Jay Hall. One Saturday night, a worried dowdy lady wandered into our dark crowded party room. We were singing "Who kicked Nelly in the Belly in the Barn." We heard a loud slap, followed by a scream, "My daughter doesn't come to places like this at fifteen!" She and the young girl were quickly escorted to the front door on 114th Street. Clearly, in addition to profuse apologies to the worried mother, action was needed. We created a subpoena validated with stamps from a silver dollar and a beer keg. The errant cradle robber was charged with corrupting the morals of a minor. He could barely handle his anxiety, wanting to make his subpoena the problem of the fraternity at large, however, without exactly telling us that he had received it. For at least two months, he wheedled to have the matter placed on the formal chapter agenda, which we refused to do. "What do you mean, Brother Dick? *We* are in what kind of trouble?"

All pledges had to work for our black cook from Harlem, John Scott. Built like a fireplug, Scotty, a short and seemingly jolly man, became an absolute tyrant in the kitchen. We dreaded these several days a week: washing dishes, setting tables, and preparing lunch and dinner meals. Scotty lost no opportunity to lord it over the white kids. One day, I had enough of it and took a swing at him. Although he was four inches shorter than I was, he quickly decked me. We then had a series of set-to's where he would laugh and "wrassle" me, as he put it, to the floor. Looking to best him somehow, I challenged him to a game of pool because, I believed, as a result of my misspent youth in Riverdale Avenue pool rooms, that I could shoot pool. We went upstairs to our pool room, where Scotty was not usually seen, and we each put ten dollars on the table. After the break, Scotty ran the whole table. My respect for this man grew and we remained friends for years. During medical school and residency, he served as a bartender for my parties. I learned something about manhood from Scotty. Once I bragged to him about teasing a girlfriend to make her jealous. Scotty's comment was, "You can't do that. There's a cock on every corner." I lost track of Scotty after about ten years. He was paid generously and all the brothers loved him. I can still smell and taste his wonderful pork chops. In spite of his sage advice to me, Scotty had chronic woman problems. A number of "wives" came to the house on 114th Street looking for him, and on these occasions, he fled the kitchen to hide in the backyard. Toward the end of lunchtime, a bookmaker came and Scotty would place bets on horseraces. We noticed that the bookie usually came about five or ten minutes after the first race at Lincoln Downs in Rhode Island had been completed. A scouting party was sent there, by train, to report by phone relay, the results of the race. The brothers then placed heavy bets on that first race which the bookie refused. He knew, judging from the size of the action, that something was fishy. Scotty was outraged, but there were no hard feelings. For a fee, the dark-suited bespectacled little man later agreed to serve our phony subpoena.

A number of members' names had the second, the third or junior after them: John J. Atkins III, William Stetson Boals II, and Frederic Warner Brewen Jr. We had to know the names of all thirty brothers by heart including their middle names. The brothers were solicitous about my cultural transformation. Some disapproved of my Bronx-style ties and gave me several good Rep ties. I was advised to shop at Brooks Brothers, but I did best at sales at S Klein's on the Square, which carried name labels if one knew what to look for. After finishing surgical residency, I bought my first Brooks Bothers suit. As freshman brothers, one of our social obligations was to escort young women to the Debutante Ball at the Plaza Hotel. I had dated a lot. I was a good dancer, and felt confident when I arrived in a rented tuxedo at the duplex on Park Avenue to pick up Alisson Grissom III. This date proved to be a disaster. A wispy blond greeted me nervously at the door. Her parents looked on suspiciously, probably wondering what kind of Fonzi was taking their daughter out. She got me out of there quickly.

We took a cab to the bar at the Biltmore Hotel on 42nd Street, the first traditional stop of the evening. Crowded into a booth with three other couples, the mission here was to order cocktails. Though I had just turned eighteen, I had plenty of experience ordering drinks favored by Bronx bars—rye and ginger, rum and coke, Seven and Seven, Stingers, Grasshoppers, and so on. What would Allison like to drink? She hesitated and fussed. The waiter, tapping his foot, grew more impatient by the second. The other couples were now staring at us. I knew that I would have to inflate the waiter's tip. I recited an endless litany of the drinks, including everything I could think of, finally offering her a beer. At last, my date loudly exclaimed, "Beer makes me fart." Italian and Irish girls in the Bronx never said anything like that. As a matter of fact, up till then, I had never heard any young woman discussing farting or admitting to it in any way. This was bad, really bad. The willowy girl was a surprisingly clumsy dancing partner, stumbling over her feet, stepping on mine and completely unable to follow a lead. Unable to erase the image of her farting from my mind, and tired of pushing her around like a truck, I suggested an early night and she readily agreed. I paid a taxi to take her home early. I was out the cost of a rented tuxedo, the drinks and the extra tip for the irritated waiter. The extra expense to pay for the cab to end that evening was well spent. I walked west crosstown on 59th Street and rode the Broadway line up to 116th Street. The senior brothers who had arranged this date were deeply concerned when the story of the Allison date filtered back to them. I explained her farting declaration, which they deemed only mildly outrageous. They took my own behavior to task. I had deeply offended obscure tribal mores, which I could not comprehend. Apparently, farting was acceptable as a topic of conversation in exalted waspy social circles.

By my second year, other cultural surprises were lying in wait. A former president of the fraternity was to marry a socialite in Pittsfield, Massachusetts. We had been invited to his wedding, but the reception was to be a totally dry Methodist affair. Crammed into a large station wagon, the brothers and their dates carried elaborately wrapped boxes during the drive north. I was not carrying a package and, halfway there, was asked about my gift. I produced a lace envelope from my inside jacket pocket with $50 enclosed for the bride. Their reaction was incredulous. I explained, "At weddings, we give money." We had to leave the highway in Connecticut where I was helped to buy a vase, elaborately wrapped to everyone's satisfaction. This gift was worth less than $50. The wedding was upscale but stuffy. I pitied the groom who had to have his drinks at his parents' house. The social life, the fraternity and the intellectual discipline of Columbia were powerful forces, but these never completely changed me. I continue to give money at weddings, citing an old Italian custom.

By sophomore year, the swimming pool at Columbia was operating, but I was not doing as well as I should have been. Working out with the current Olympic backstroke champion, Allen Stack, I was always a body length behind him. Allen was about six foot four and had big hands; I was short and had small hands. The coach thought that I was never going to go any faster and suggested that I take up diving. I did, but after hitting my head on the board, I was never able to execute a gainer with a score over five. After a long workout, Allen asked casually, "Ralph, I hear you are doing very well in school. What are your plans?" I said that I had planned to study physics, but was now considering medical school. Allen, a student at Kent Law School, told me that the only reason he had been admitted to Columbia, with his C average from Yale, was because he was an Olympic champion. He thought that I might be better off concentrating on premedical studies. I was growing further and further apart from my colleagues in physics.

They were brilliant and kind, but some were more creative mathematical thinkers than I would ever be. Although I could still get A's without studying much, it seemed clear that many of my classmates would go much further than I would in mathematical reasoning. Those more interested in laboratory work seemed to have inwardly turned personalities. I understood how absorbing laboratory work could be, but these men were boring and I was lonely among them.

Premedical students seemed to be a bit more compatible, though a few were grubby characters that roamed about anxiously spying out on each other's grades. Their lot on the Columbia campus was a fierce competition for grades without a trace of intellectual curiosity or pleasure. Premedical students in Beta Theta Pi were agreeable and well rounded. Taking an active interest in my future, Gilbert Highet had me write extra essays. When I described my career plan, which was to study high polymer physics to delineate interacting forces within long polymers as they stretched and bent, Highet looked puzzled. "What are you going to do with that Ralph, make a stickier adhesive?" He assigned, as summer reading, Somerset Maugham's *Of Human Bondage*, Flaubert's *Salammbo* and *Madame Bovary*. He also suggested Kohler's *Behavior of Apes* and Sheldon on *The Varieties of Temperament*. Highet's words about stickier adhesive kept floating up in my mind, even as I read Sheldon's psychological psuedoscience, which I did find interesting. By the end of my second year, I had decided to apply for medical school.

In second year, the Department of Psychology indoctrinated us in "health sciences," a sex course featuring Stone and Stone's *A Marriage Manual*. The lubricious and highly specific details in this graphic book led to more experimentation. This new expertise might or might not have been a good thing. We were horny enough as it was. The teacher, a Professor Malffotto, preached situational ethics and plastic morals, all disguised in a kind of bland affability. Just like the freshman English professor, he seemed interested in the students' personal lives and asked for an essay about a sexual experience. I concocted an outrageous story from Freud's

Psychopathology about fantasies of falling in love and doing things with chickens. He immediately called me for a conference, and to my surprise, he was unfamiliar with Freud's writings about this fetish. I had thought he would recognize my essay as a tongue-in-cheek prank. Instead, he was furious. I wrote him off as another creep, like the English instructor who wanted a similar essay. My sense of Catholic Puritanism remained even though its religious basis had temporarily fled. Father Barry, the pastor at St. John's, appeared in my mind to be a more honorable character than Malfotto. I would have enjoyed seeing these two debate moral issues. The priest would have won hands down.

The final examination in "health" yielded my only career C. We were asked to consider the problems of a Columbia freshman coming from a town in the Midwest. He became quite ill adjusted. He missed his family, could not sleep, was failing academically, and was masturbating obsessively, "which bothered him a great deal since this was against his *particular* religion." What were our recommendations? Obviously, he should have immediately consulted a member of the psychology department. I opened the blue book gleefully and started to write. I suggested that he go out for football or crew, preferably football. Coach Little might make a man of him. He should pledge to a fraternity, if one would have him, and start dating Barnard girls. If he really wanted to get laid, he could go downtown to the dance halls. He could find a religion that encouraged masturbation. Hinduism came to mind. But, at that moment, I was not certain. Further research in tantric sex was required. Malffotto was not amused. I had a lot of fun writing the essay and I would have failed had I not answered the objective part of the exam completely correctly. Knowing what I know now, this young person in this case was seriously depressed. But I remain certain that talking to the senior member of that psychology department would have made him worse. Today, there would be a consultative talk and psychotropic drugs to help the lonely young man over the initial hurdles of college life

Professor Polycarp Kusch advised me against a career change from physics to medicine. He was disappointed and thought I was doing well in physics, but my heart was not really in this work. Professor Kusch sent me to see the dean of the college, who insisted that I take an aptitude test before making a decision. The dean appeared puzzled after reviewing the results of that examination. "Well, you are best suited to be a musician. Do you play a musical instrument?" I did play the ukulele and liked irregular hours and entertainment, but I could not figure out how this test determined suitability for medicine. The dean was kind enough to enlighten me. One of the key questions was: "Would you like to have a monkey as a pet?" Having observed monkeys hurling turds at unwary tourists in the Central Park Zoo, I had marked, categorically never. But this question was included to elicit a sense of caring. Presumably, if you liked monkeys, you ought to like people. As the results of the test were equivocal, the dean consented to my change to premedical studies.

Years later, as a faculty member on a medical school admissions committee, I was struck by the insistence that desirable candidates should have "bedpan experience." Working in an Alzheimer's nursing home or caring for the criminally insane was highly regarded by a certain element. Clearly, one must be caring to be a good doctor. Sick people, above all else, require competence, constant availability and long, hardworking hours. Unavailability at night and on weekends paralleled exactly the expressed humanism of "socially oriented" faculty, mostly psychiatrists or "family practitioners." These were exactly the ones insisting on "bedpan experience."

Once I got permission to change my major, I immediately started organic chemistry. Medical schools accepted only one in five applicants at that time and an A in organic chemistry was a virtual prerequisite for acceptance. The ability to handle the Grignard reagent, to memorize the massive formulae of organic chemistry, and the ability to synthesize organic compounds in the laboratory were important elements for a successful medical school application. In some degree, the ability to work well in the laboratory might have had validity, for a medical career. My laboratory partner was a man named Delaney, my alphabetical predecessor. We became experts at synthesizing complex ethers, working cooperatively rather than competitively. We both became surgeons and we both enjoyed the hands on laboratory work. The last two years of college merged into one frantic year. Without taking the classes, I read for the remaining requirements of graduation, and passed with the required B plus to exercise "professional option." This allowed me to enter medical school after my junior year. During this year, my childhood friend, Dan Ryan, from the old neighborhood, neglected his diabetes and grew sicker and sicker. He died that fall. His final gesture of friendship was to sell me a 1941 Plymouth for ten dollars. This was more a gift than a sale. The body of the old sedan was a wreck, with wired-on fenders and taped-in headlights, but the car ran beautifully, provided I fiddled with the voltage regulator periodically. I used it for work and during my first year of medical school.

The medical school interviewer at New York University asked, "Will you get an A in organic chemistry?" I replied, "Yes." Doctors Sherwood Lawrence and Sol Farber both nodded their heads. I was accepted. During the interview, I had told them sincere and truthful things about wanting to help people and being a humanitarian. Alvin Levine, a pale-faced Hasidic Jewish boy from Brooklyn, was also at that interview. Al looked like Jerry Seinfeld and had the same offbeat sense of humor. He was brilliant, quietly cynical, and honest. During his interview, laughter emanated from the room. Al had told them, in response to the usual why-do-you-want-to-be-a-doctor question: "I want to be a doctor so I can be rich and drive a big black Cadillac." The committee was impressed with his answer. He had such a comical way putting it that it was hard to take him seriously. Of course, he also had the highest grade point average in the city of New York. Toward the end of medical school, I learned that Al was first in the class and that I was second. We were never told our grades or our rank until the very end of senior year. After all, who wants a doctor who is in the lower half of the class? I was hoping for an exalted internship. However, Al told me that he was going into dermatology. His goal was to open an office in each of the five boroughs of New York.

Somehow, I feel I didn't learn everything as well as I should have during those years. Radical changes were required to make a Bronx boy into an Ivy League collegian. I recognized, years later, that the process had not been completed. I thought about my encounter with real lions. Getting my full attention required a great deal of noise, but even lions, really, do not roar when they talk. Perhaps, they only roar when baited, and then it will be too late. They make themselves known by quiet "woof woofs" in descending crescendos. I left the Columbia Lion with no parting words. I did not take time to attend graduation, and after the first year of medical school, my *cum laude* diploma arrived by mail. The balance of the Regent's scholarship partially paid for tuition for the first year of medical school, so I had to keep working. We children of the Depression were terrified of being in debt. I left the quiet lion, having learned a better way to live and for that, I was grateful. I wish that I taken time to listen more attentively and at least for another year.

MEDICINE, THE MISTRESS

*I swear by Apollo, Physician, and Ascelapius and Hygieia
and Panaceia and all the gods and goddesses . . .*
The Physicians Oath

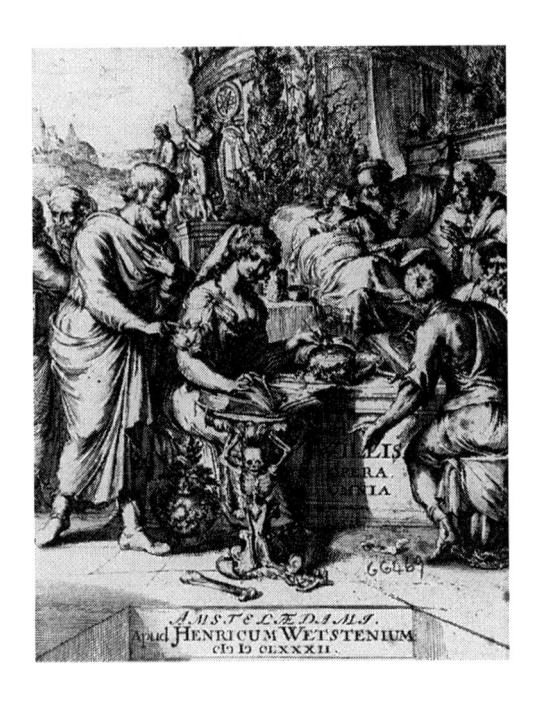

**Aesculapius and Hygeia, Courtesy of the
National Library of Medicine**

I met the love of my life at twenty-one years of age, when I began my studies at New York University School of Medicine. I left the crystalline certainty of physics for a life-long affair with a bewildering mistress. Gilbert Highet, the Anthon Professor of Greek and Latin at Columbia, encouraged this choice. Medicine, and later surgery, became my life and proved exceptionally rewarding. The disadvantages of the relationship became obvious only later, and related to jealousy and rancor among suitors who were pledged to a supposedly altruistic calling, inordinate demands for time and attention, and an ever-changing persona. Medicine, the mistress, proved to be fickle in some ways as I embraced a curious and changing mixture of art, anecdote and science. Then, later, powerful financial forces competed for her attention. I discovered her defects bit by bit, as often happens, after years of intimacy, when it became too late to turn back.

Upon acceptance to medical school, I had to leave Manhattan, giving up a cozy fifth-floor room at the Beta House, and move to my mother's house in Yonkers to begin commuting once again. Italians have a name for bachelors who live with their mothers. They call them "vitelloni," or little veal calves. Vitelloni hide behind mother's skirts, and though admittedly ignominious, the arrangement has its advantages over other alternatives. A girlfriend, a couple of years older than I, wanted me to marry her just after I had been accepted to medical school. We went to midnight mass one Christmas and the next morning, she drove me back to Kimball Avenue in her new Pontiac and made this astonishing proposal. When I refused to even discuss it, she threatened to talk to my mother. I warned her that an old-fashioned Italian lady would not likely welcome a woman, older than I, demanding to marry her son because they had slept together. I left her sitting in the car, which remained across the street for what seemed to be an eternity. Then, she left. Vitelloni can live shamelessly and comfortably, coming and going as they please, and evading marriage. I cared for this woman, but I sensed that the combination of medicine and her demands would be more than I could handle.

A fellow student, who lived in the Bronx, and I drove to Gun Hill Road station in my rickety 1941 Plymouth six days a week. On Saturday mornings, we were treated to conferences during which we saw patients. We boarded the Third Avenue elevated train, which shook and rumbled down to East 23rd Street. The antiquated buildings of the medical school on First Avenue from 26th to 28th Street faced the massive walls of Bellevue Hospital, a three-block walk from the elevated station.

When we returned to Gun Hill Road at night, the decrepit sedan, with its wired-on fenders, was always exactly where we left it. This might not happen in the Bronx today.

For the first time in my life, I studied assiduously. We read *Gray's Anatomy* on the morning train and biochemistry on the jolting ride back to Gun Hill Road in the Bronx. Then, I drove to the Kimball Avenue home, and studied until midnight. This grinding cycle continued for three months. Biochemistry and anatomy comprised the entire first trimester. When I could recognize minor mistakes or inconsistencies in the textbooks, I knew I had mastered the material. I studied all the time, except for Saturday nights which were reserved for small revels such as dancing and dating. I rose at noon on Sunday and read till bedtime. We assimilated an enormous amount of information and learned an entirely new vocabulary. In spite of its drudgery, the total immersion was stimulating. We were being initiated into a secret and arcane society. In 1952, the lay public knew very little about medicine. Our curricular schedule was simple. Formal lectures were then confined to an hour in the mornings. The medical faculty knew then what we have forgotten today: lectures are not a good means of adult education. We did things in anatomy, biochemistry, and later, in physiology laboratories during that first year. The approach was labor intensive for us and for the faculty, and instructors were always in attendance. Autobiography is not, nor should it be, a template for modern medical education, but my first year of medical school was much more fun than the seven hours of lecture a day which current medical students endure.

Gross anatomy consumed two-thirds of our freshman year. We dissected our leathery formaldehyde-soaked cadavers and studied histology with newly purchased microscopes. Mine, which I still have, is an antique monocular scope with a powerful double condenser that draws in light from any source. Later, I spent much of my life operating on blood vessels supplying the lower extremity, and, coincidentally, my first medical school dissection involved these vessels and nerves in Scarpa's triangle, an area defined by the muscles and ligaments in the upper thigh. Anatomic zones and structures were named for the courageous Renaissance Italian anatomists who performed human dissections, even though they had been forbidden to do so by the church. Their names are intriguing, but few students now bother to learn anatomic eponyms. I hold them dear because they symbolize knowledge so perilously wrested from the constrictions of the Medieval mind. That knowledge was as important for those times and up to the nineteenth century and well into my time in medical school as molecular biology and the genetic code have now become in these years. While we dissected and learned gross anatomy, we also peered at and memorized the details of cells and tissues. We knew nothing about the intricate details of cells and fine structure, which linked biochemistry and physiology to the functions of these cells. That came much later when the electron microscope, delayed in its development by Hitler in World War II, came to be used. Years later, I had the opportunity to examine changes in cellular structure in response to hemorrhage and infection. In the 1950s, we mistakenly believed the number of chromosomes to be forty-eight. Two decades later, when I should have known better, I had this belief sharply corrected by an amused genetics professor.

Professor Joseph Pick, a Viennese anatomist and an expert on the autonomic nervous system, was my first instructor. He was an intense and terrifyingly single-minded man. He felt that anatomy was the most important of our studies as future doctors. He said, "The human body was the instrument that we would play for the rest of our lives. We needed to understand its most intimate details." We took his admonition seriously. On one occasion, in stripping a flimsy outer layer from the femoral artery, Pick asked, "Do you think this makes any difference in life?" I impulsively replied, "It doesn't look like much, it probably does not." He stared at me disapprovingly through his bespectacled loupes. He was writing a book on the enervation of vessels. This, clearly, was not the right answer.

Later, his book helped me perform nerve-sparing vascular reconstructions to prevent or treat impotence or male erectile dysfunction. These procedures involved limiting vascular dissection and sparing nerves intimately associated with some of the large abdominal arteries. At that time, I had no idea that I was to become a surgeon. My partner had announced that he was to be a surgeon, but Pick became highly critical of his anatomic preparations. This student's dissection technique was awful, and his fumbling did not escape notice. Staring heavenward, he would pick and poke delicate structures, all the while never looking at the field of dissection. Pick, after inspecting his first serious effort, said in a thick German accent, "Ach, it looks like the rats have been gnawing here." This comment threw the budding surgeon into a deep depression: he later became an internist. I too got to the point where I could not bear to watch while he dissected, and left to study *Grant's Atlas* in an anteroom. At that stage of my life, I doubted that I would ever have the capability or skill to become a surgeon, although Pick grudgingly acknowledged my handiwork as "not bad."

My dissecting partner was a good-hearted person and became, I am sure, a fine doctor. As the product of a Catholic high school and college education, his beliefs were sincere and heartfelt. But we clashed continually and mainly over religion. He had not been exposed to or read original sources. Jesuits had, in the course of his education, inculcated particular views and censored others. Some of this might have simply been part of his peculiarly dogmatic intellect. We became involved in curious, long-winded, and unproductive arguments. He had an annoying way of provoking me into taking a stand on some issue or another, then shaking his head woefully from side to side saying, "No, oh, no" to my secular or irreverent views which I often made more extreme just to provoke him. Whether citing philosophy or his version of a fact, I believed him to be mostly wrong. But some of our dialogues were helpful in crystallizing issues related to our studies. We traveled together during our first year of medical school. I was not as tactful or kind as I should have been and this remains as one of my major failings. By my second year, I found more compatible companions in the medical school's class who did not chide me for my secular viewpoints and my status as a fallen-away Catholic. Years later, I found this comment by a senior surgeon to a search committee, "He tolerates fools poorly." As I had already become a chair of surgery, I took this comment as a compliment. I now understand that this is not a compliment, and over the years, I tried to become more tolerant. Though in some ways, I felt that mistress medicine would also not tolerate fools gladly.

We used *Cunningham's Dissection Manual* as well as *Gray's Anatomy*. We, therefore, memorized both English and Latin anatomic terms and argued pedantically over proper nomenclature. I met a lively Irish girl, a former medical student from Belfast, who convinced me to use English nomenclature and I was intrigued with her. The events prompting her departure from Ireland and medical school and the reasons she lived on Long Island with an aunt and uncle remained murky. I never found out as much about her or understood her, as I should have. I was preoccupied with my own concerns. We had wonderful dissolute weekends on Long Island and in Westchester and things went well until the issue of marriage arose. I was not ready to marry. She stayed with me until the night of her departure to the United Kingdom to marry an older man. I became physically ill for weeks after she left. I experienced constant nausea and lost ten pounds before recovering. But I was lucky. I learned from this experience why Italians place three coffee beans in a goblet of Galliano to remind us that love, sex, and marriage are three different things.

Freshman medical school pranks in anatomy class compensated for the horrific sight of rows of human bodies stretched out on tables in the sky-lit dissecting room. No one fainted or became ill. Our introduction to the naked human body by Dr. Joseph Odiorne was gentle and respectful. Apocryphal rumors circulated in the city that a human arm had been found hanging on a subway strap during rush hour. No one at NYU was responsible, but we were warned formally that desecration of a human body would be severely punished. In spite of such warnings, irreverent pranks did occur. A massive cadaver erection greeted our four female students one morning as they uncovered their wrinkled corpse. Early that morning, an unnamed student had injected its penile cavernous bodies with saline, under pressure. Similarly induced artificial erections are now used clinically to diagnose and correct male erectile dysfunction with drugs.

We also implanted a small white wooden egg deep into the vaginal vault of one of the three female cadavers. The four male students assigned to this female were supposed to share so that thirty-five students, all male, could learn about female anatomy. At that time, many men really had not had a good look at female genitalia. Experience was limited to gropes in the dark or to diagrams. Ingram Kerner, later known as "Ingrown," and his three associates who owned this cadaver, were remarkably selfish; they guarded her anatomic secrets jealously. During a formal demonstration of vaginal examination, observed by all and supervised by a grave senior instructor, Ingrown poked and fumbled within the vagina for what seemed like an interminable time. He finally extracted the small white object, which appeared to be a robin's egg. With a look of pure astonishment, he myopically turned the object over and over just under his nose. After a long moment, a chicken-like cackle sounded from the back of the gathering. Collapsing with laughter, I actually fell to the floor, drenching my slacks in the ubiquitous pools of formaldehyde. The formaldehyde odor permeated our persons during our long months of gross anatomy. On the subway, a fellow medical student could be recognized by a characteristic smell and a preoccupied facial expression.

During biochemistry, we were assigned to measure the chemical component excreted in our own daily urine output. We lugged gallon jars through the New York Public Transit system to find out how much nitrogen, urea, and ammonia our urine contained. We, also, were required to analyze the protein, fat and carbohydrate contents of an egg down to the last milligram. I still recall all of these values to this day. At one crucial point in my life, during my surgical board's oral examination, Dr. Robert M Zollinger asked me to recite the caloric content and the composition of an egg. I reeled off 80 to 100 calories depending on size and 150 milligrams of cholesterol depending on feed. He stopped me before I got to protein and lecithin. He, then, abruptly asked how much a milliequivalent of chloride ion weighed. The atomic weight of 35 emerged from somewhere in the depths of my brain where freshman chemistry lived. He blurted out, "What are you, a wise guy?" He dismissed me without further questions or comments. Dr. Zollinger was reputed to be a terrifying examiner. I found out later that these were his favorite questions. On one occasion, another hapless examinee walked into the room, and, seeing Zollinger, promptly vomited. Zollinger glowered at the yellow-green pool on the floor and said, "Tell me what's in it and I'll pass you."

We did physiology in the ancient 26th Street laboratory, now long gone, across the street from Bellevue. We used smoked recording drums and struggled to keep our animals alive to obtain meaningful data. Gradually, I became the team member designated to do cut downs, insert pressure monitors and to maintain an airway in the heavily anesthetized dogs or cats. We performed a classic experiment, stimulating the vagal nerves in the beating and exposed heart of a frog to observe the heartbeat slowing, as acetylcholine flowed from the nerve endings. Then we added a minute amount of saline solution and transferred the pericardial fluid into the pericardial sac of another exposed frog heart. Immediately, the second heart slowed as well, indicating the presence of a soluble neurochemical mediator released by the vagal nerves. Dr. Otto Loewe, who had won the Nobel Prize for this discovery, tottered about the laboratory, scrutinizing each of our preparations and nodding approvingly, "Ah-ha, you find der Vagustuff." The physiology faculty had arranged this special occasion. The greatness of an Otto Loewe seemed almost within our grasp. The physiology lecturers were stellar, particularly Homer Smith, on renal physiology. In his laboratory, we drank gallons of water and measured our renal clearances of solutes. We had to produce urine hourly and half hourly to get the experiment right, and some of us found this to be very difficult. Dr. Smith confided to us that his concept of urinary solute clearance, so evident on the surface, had taken him years to figure out. His candor was comforting; we had difficulty in grasping the concept during our three months of study. During bacteriology, McLeod and associates lectured us about viral transfer, phage, and DNA. With Avery, Mcleod had discovered the DNA transforming principle, but a qualifying phrase that the transforming factor might be a contaminant—a waffle insisted upon by an internal Rockefeller Institute reviewer—at the end of their classic paper, cost them the Nobel Prize. At the end of a brilliant exposition, they hedged, suggesting that the powerful mucoid residue that they had discovered might not be actually what they had so clearly demonstrated it to be.

A tall, silver-haired man elegantly dressed in a dark three-piece suit greeted us on our first day of medical school. He was a prominent Park Avenue rheumatologist and the dean of the medical school. He reassured us that the faculty intended that we should all succeed. We would not know our grades unless we had a problem. He was a practicing doctor, and appeared quite successful, but he admitted that all he could do for arthritis was to advise hot paraffin soaks and aspirin. He told us that the future, in our hands, might offer more. He described, with great enthusiasm, work being done at NYU on the biochemistry of DNA by Dr. Severo Ochoa, who later won a Nobel Prize. McKewen bred hybrid daylilies, and I later planted some daylilies that bore his name. This impressive figure said that, in contrast to college studies, everything taught in medical school would be of use. Some of us took him literally and there was much to learn.

By the time third-year clinical clerkships at Bellevue began, I conceded that it might be impossible to learn everything. While reading large clinical textbooks from cover to cover, I soon forgot basic science. My ephemeral mistress was much more intricate than could be imagined. Some of us puzzled over exactly how much we had to know. My classmate, Ralph Cavalieri, and I cornered the Nobelist Andre Cournand, famed for his catheterization work, in a small cluttered laboratory in the basement of Bellevue Hospital. Cournand and his colleague, Richards, were renowned for having passed a catheter from his arm into the chambers of the heart. He was puttering about in his laboratory. We asked, "What do we have to learn?" He turned, looked at us curiously, pulled the collar of his white coat up about his neck, and scurried from the room saying over his shoulder, "Everything, everything." So, some of us did try to learn everything.

Summers were free, so some fortunate students could take laboratory electives. But I had to work. I served as a lifeguard for several summers; this was pleasant and glamorous work, with plenty of girls to meet. But it paid poorly. Luckily, I got a job moving steel for a new bridge on the Hutchinson Parkway. This labor paid six dollars an hour, an incredible amount of money for those times. Courtesy of the Teamsters Union and the International Union of Hod Carriers and Laborers, I got through medical school without having to borrow money. I have saved those old union cards in an old wallet that I still keep in a bureau drawer. Though I lived at home and commuted, I still partied on weekends with my fraternity brothers at Columbia but gradually grew more distant from them as well. Once again, I left old friends behind. My medical studies demanded full attention.

Young people should not rush into careers or courtships. My truncated experience in college followed by the first and second year of medical school contributed to a certain immaturity and impatience. Leisure and time are needed to develop political and social skills. Scholars, laboring in isolation, do not develop the skills needed to tolerate individual idiosyncrasies or to understand group dynamics. The demands of medicine in those times may have led some of us into unrecognized solipsism, an extreme form of individual idealism, which might account for later troubles in personal relationships. A senior year at Columbia would have helped me immensely. Later, I needed to develop leadership skills and tolerance in assuming responsibilities for others. Early, I was entranced with the vastness of medicine, and, in trying to learn everything, I became impatient with myself and sometimes became unduly harsh with others.

During third year, I made a lucky diagnosis, establishing clinical reputation of sorts among colleagues and faculty. An anxious, frail and neurotic-appearing woman presented to the surgical service at Bellevue complaining of weakness, fatigue and vomiting. She spoke Polish and some Spanish. I was able to get her history using elementary Spanish. Her serum sodium was low and potassium, a little high. She complained that her skin was growing dark. Then her husband remarked that, when kissed, she tasted salty to him. These refugees from Poland had migrated to Spain to enter the United States after an arduous dangerous journey. During these travels, she had acquired tuberculosis, involving her spine and the back muscles. A cascade of calcification within the sheath of the psoas muscle and collapsed vertebra signaled this old and now inactive infection.

Because of her vomiting, the surgical service admitted her as a case of gallbladder disease. This did not seem to be a case of gallbladder disease at all; she exhibited no abdominal signs. I looked up all possible causes of vomiting, low sodium, and darkened skin in French's *Index of Differential Diagnosis*, a useful volume still on my shelf. The confluence of symptoms and signs spelled out Addison's disease, an adrenal insufficiency due to the destruction of her adrenal glands by tuberculosis, causing her to excrete salt in excess. The surgical residents were too busy to listen to an excited junior student calling them from Yonkers with arcane revelations. That night, I drove from Yonkers to Manhattan in the old Plymouth. Early the next morning, another medical student and I did a Keppler-Power water tolerance test, drawing blood and urine for electrolytes and running the specimens to the laboratory. I was a nuisance, but the residents let us proceed, and busy laboratory technicians were kind enough to help third-year students. Her test was dramatically positive. Her handling of salt and water were diagnostic of Addison's disease. It took a while, though, to convince the surgical staff that her vomiting might be due to adrenal insufficiency. The endocrinologists confirmed the diagnosis, and treated her with steroids, and her vomiting stopped. I was proud of this patient and saw her intermittently as she wended her way through Bellevue Clinic's maze.

She needed continual reassurance because of her lack of English and her terror over deportation with the diagnosis of tuberculosis. Luckily, I was able to communicate with her in Spanish. During my senior year, a fellow student told me that she had been admitted to the hospital once again. I found her cowering in the corner of a dark locked psychiatric ward. She complained to an emergency room resident that a worm had come out of her nose. This was taken as a hallucination, so she was admitted to an acute psychiatric ward. The Bellevue psychiatric wards were like a vision of hell. No one actually checked to see if there was actually a worm or what the worm looked like. Her agitated husband brought me an *Ascaris* worm, about ten inches long in a jam jar. We ceremoniously presented this worm, well pickled in alcohol, to the admitting psychiatrist. He grudgingly discharged her but admonished me that he still thought her to be deranged. His comment was accurate, given her endocrine disorder, which is known to produce mental changes, her past hardships, and her uncertain future. Thinking about my diagnosis now, the vomiting prompting the surgical admission might also have been due to worm infestation, so I had not been so clever after all.

During my senior year, I was chosen to become one of the *New York Times* "interns." This position involved sleeping in the building to attend to the urgent needs of the workforce of the newspaper at night during production of the morning edition. Here, I first encountered alcoholic fits or convulsions. Many of the *Times* newspapermen drank heavily in the nearby bars across the *Times* building and along Eighth Avenue. Drinking, I was told, was the custom among newspapermen, and, in contrast to most occupations, this was accepted behavior. When the final edition was complete, they slept during the day to return late in the afternoon to produce the next edition. During my first night on duty, I saw three convulsions or "alcoholic fits" and two cases of appendicitis, which I referred to St. Clare's Hospital. These actually both turned out to be appendicitis. The medical director, a clever internist, initially worried that his fourth-year student was overreacting. When I sent a third case that turned out to be appendicitis, the chief of surgery at St. Clare's, Dr. Robert Madden, took the time to call me to compliment me on these accurate diagnoses and also to reassure my boss.

Whenever I took a new position, clinical challenges seemed to surface with unusual frequency. The *Times* clinic was quiet until just after midnight when emergencies would appear. Some elective cases also came, after treating one of the announcers on the classic radio station, WQXR. Each announcer came for regular throat sprays in the early evening. They were peasant, entertaining men and always sober in contrast to the reporters or editors who usually smelled of alcohol. Minor complaints were easily handled, but some were certainly outside my scope of practice. The clinic had a dental chair, and one afternoon, the dentist taught me to insert temporary fillings. Night after night, workmen would appear with toothaches. I treated these with temporary fillings, and instructed them to see a dentist as soon as possible. Once the temporary filling was inserted and the pain relieved, dental care was usually neglected until my filling fell out. A particular chronic offender reappeared four times, usually at 2 or 3 A.M. I finally solved his recurring dental problem by laying out our dental tools on a tray under his nose, but this time, I included a menacing pair of pliers. When he noticed these on the tray, I suggested that, maybe, we needed to pull that tooth out. He said he liked my fillings, thanked me, and promised to see a real dentist.

The *Times* internship was just the beginning of many years of night and holiday duties, but it also offered my first taste of independence and the ability to exercise judgment. At that time, my partner and I worked alternate weekends. My wife brought

Thanksgiving and Christmas dinners from Yonkers to the *Times*, which we warmed and ate in the deserted clinic. We had married in the fall of my senior year and these were the first of many holiday dinners spent away from home. Fortunately, we were able to do this together, but there were many years when we could not. The mistress had just begun her demands.

New York University School of Medicine had a special flavor because of its municipal hospital affiliation. The patients on the wards of Bellevue were poor and humble, but the medical students and residents were devoted to them, and the patients, by and large, returned this allegiance. As their doctors, we did everything we could to care for them. Attending physicians rarely appeared on the Bellevue wards. We learned a great deal but we could have done better with more supervision. The major concern of my very first patient on the medical ward was that his Social Security check be cashed so that he could pay his landlord and not lose his apartment. Mr. Perez, a frail, dark-skinned Puerto Rican with kidney failure because of a neglected enlarged prostate, was waiting for urological surgery while a catheter drained his flaccid bladder. I did my first vena punctures on his small veins, and I felt clumsy, but he was always gracious about my inexperience. Mr. Perez lived in mortal terror of losing his small apartment, and I asked Social Service to manage his concern involving his Social Security check. A flighty, unattractive young woman spouted psychobabble and regulations at length: finally telling me that she could not or would not be able to perform this simple task. I took his check to the liquor store across the street each month, cashed it and paid the small fee. His landlord then came to his bedside to pick up the cash. It took the surgical service three months to perform his prostate operation.

We did all the blood counts and urine analyses for our patients, and ran miles to the central laboratory to type and cross-match blood for transfusions. The accuracy of the type and cross-match was our own responsibility. As the elevators were impossibly slow, we moved about the massive complex by running up and down stairs. I contracted infectious hepatitis on the Pediatric Infectious

Disease Unit during an outbreak of "black measles," a combination of measles and hepatitis. The combined processes caused jaundice and a terrifying hemorrhagic rash. These critically ill children required close contact, and it was easy to become contaminated in spite of hand washing and precautions. At that time, we never used rubber gloves as we do now. The gesture of donning gloves, now so common, would have seemed heartless. My presenting complaint was an inability to run up and down stairs. I was slumped against the wall, resting in a stairwell when a medical resident, also running the stairs, paused briefly to say, "Hey, Ralph, you are jaundiced."

Dr. Saul Farber, then a medical attending, poked at my enlarged tender liver, warned me not to drink any alcohol at all, and sent me home to rest. My wife cooked me a steak and I holed up in our apartment on McLean Avenue in the Bronx, reading textbooks, and eating well during the last weeks of my senior year. The fatigue disappeared quickly, but Dr. Farber was worried because I continued to have a slightly elevated bilirubin level. This turned out to be a chemical finding due to a harmless congenital abnormality later diagnosed as Gilbert's disease. Rather than delaying my internship, I reported to Columbia Presbyterian Hospital on July 1. I felt fine.

Dr. Farber, an avuncular saint, later served as dean at New York University until 1998, when New York University merged with Mt. Sinai. During my second year, I visited him complaining of a headache. He was working in his laboratory, juggling tubes of mysterious liquids as I described my complaint. He glanced at me intently and said, "You know, working up a headache is a complex thing." I said, "Yes." "Are you under stress?" "Of course." He took a blood pressure cuff and stethoscope from a drawer, to check my pulse and blood pressure. These, he told me, were normal. "Maybe you should slack off a little and take aspirin; it will probably go away." It did. This contradicts the axiom warning that every headache should be considered a brain tumor until proven otherwise. There would have been little to do, at that time, about a brain tumor in any event. A psychiatrist of that era had treated

Irving Berlin before his brain tumor was diagnosed. An aneurysm might have been a different matter, but at that time, even this would have been quite a surgical challenge. On the other hand, one of my favorite residents used to say, "Never look for something you don't want to find." Our reflex response today would be to order a CAT scan.

Dr. Herbert Kaden, a young masterful cardiologist, taught physical diagnosis. Dressed in our best shirts and ties, we carried starched white coats, took an uptown train to the 59th Street Bridge, walked halfway across and then rode an elevator down to Goldwater Hospital, on an island in the middle of the East River. We had been instructed to dress well for these occasions, "You are doctors, not dockworkers," said Elaine Ralley, one of our clinical preceptors. Under Kaden's supervision, we examined chronic cardiac patients with well-characterized heart murmurs. These old men, also subjects for the board examinations in internal medicine, were happy to have us practice on them, and dropped helpful hints about their murmurs. On my very first visit, I was lucky enough to detect an aortic valvular insufficiency due to syphilis. Dr. Kaden, an enthusiastic teacher who stimulated my lifelong interest in examining patients, was pleased with this performance. He had pioneered the use of procainamide for the control of cardiac arrhythmias, a tricky business in those days and even today when we use continuous monitoring devices. Residents treated patients admitted to our cardiology ward and, as seniors, we sat by the bedside to monitor the pulse rate and blood pressure as these intravenous drugs were injected with great caution. The discipline of continued intense observation taught us a great deal about the clinical course of acutely ill patients.

Senior year passed rapidly. Because I felt weakest in pediatrics, I took an elective in infectious disease with Dr. Saul Krugman. We treated victims of an outbreak of varicella amongst Puerto Rican immigrants, a terrible disease in young adults. In contrast to the benign course of childhood chicken pox, the disease in adolescence caused a lethal pneumonia that appeared radiographically much like miliary tuberculosis. In spite of its viral etiology, we learned that antibiotics were absolutely required. Tetracycline seemed to work best. Now, I think that this might have been due to the peculiar anti-inflammatory effects of that drug rather than its characteristics as an antibiotic. My bout with hepatitis cut this interesting experience short.

The fourth-year surgical elective with Dr. Rousselot at St. Vincent's Hospital in Greenwich Village changed my career plans. Up until this time, I had planned on becoming an internist. Regrettably, I told the chief of surgery at Bellevue, kindly Dr Mullholland, that I wanted internal medicine because, "Internists think." He chuckled tolerantly and replied, "Do you think surgeons do not?" As far as I could see, unsupervised surgical residents at Bellevue did not think much, and their surgical results were sometimes disasters. The axiom, "See one, do one, teach one," led, in my opinion, to intolerably poor results. Much, much later, as an educator, I was to get an opportunity to improve things, but I am not sure that I did as well with this as I could have, though I really tried to watch over everything my residents did. At St. Vincent's, the chief of surgery seemed to have a handle on everything that was going on, and attending surgeons were much in evidence. The sisters ran the hospital with a caring but stern discipline befitting the care of the sick. The only time I saw their equanimity falter was when the poet, Dylan Thomas presented with delirium and in florid liver failure, and then, wife and mistress appeared at his bedside. While he raved obscenely, the two women screamed imprecations at each other. We listened from the hall as the sisters abandoned the field. The poet died within hours. This scene was an exception. Observing firsthand the fine surgical residents and the clinical results at this hospital, I decided on surgical internship.

As promised by Dean McKewen, we never received our medical school grades until the very end, when we needed to apply for internships. I guessed that I was probably doing well, but was not sure of my standing. The only grade I did learn about was in anatomy. My wife, a graduate anatomy student, had access to these grades. We had both scored in the nineties, but her score was higher than mine. The dean met with each of us at the end of senior year to counsel us on internship selection. I then learned that I was second in our class of 145 students. I asked who was first. It was Al Levine, who had said from the start that he would become a dermatologist. Internships at the Brigham or the Massachusetts General did not interest him. He chose a classy private hospital in Westchester, with on call duty every fifth night.

Dean Hubbard requested that seniors take a voluntary "aptitude test" for medicine for an educational study. I recognized the same psychology aptitude test I had encountered during college, which at the time, determined that I was best suited to be a musician or entertainer. With experience in recognizing its intrinsic biases, I identified the touchy-feely questions and replied to these positively. All questions about monkeys, terrible, filthy, vicious creatures, were answered in the strongest affirmative. I now absolutely loved monkeys. Even after years of experimental work with vascular diseases using subhuman primates, I could not recommend a monkey as a pet. The dean later marveled that I had gotten one of the highest aptitudes for medicine ever recorded for that test. I think it impossible to determine who might, or who might not, make a good doctor or contribute richly to the profession. Great doctors seem to come in all shapes, sizes and temperaments, and, solipsism aside, they are mostly smart and love their work inordinately.

Eve and I took a Greyhound Bus tour in midwinter of senior year to interview for internships. Remembering this exhausting journey, my heart goes out to senior medical students who appear for interview in the dead of winter. Most are searching for the best possible training. Wearing their hearts on their sleeves, they incur expenses that most of them can ill-afford. We rode the bus all the way to Indiana and stopped in several cities on the way back. I had considered practicing among Midwesterners, having roomed with an amiable fraternity brother, a Hoosier, who I admired for his relaxed and kindly demeanor. I decided against Indiana when I saw a surgical resident changing a perineal wound dressing with an unlit cigar in his mouth. I interviewed in Detroit where they offered a mixed internship in both medicine and surgery, at Presbyterian Hospital in New York, the University of Michigan and at Western Reserve in Cleveland. It was an exhausting bus trip. I believe I might have selected Western Reserve, but that did not happen for some years. Eve got a call from Presbyterian letting us know that I would be listed first there. So I ranked Columbia Presbyterian first, staying in New York in familiar surroundings. Later, I needed to leave New York City to pursue mistress medicine in other places. Love affairs are irrational and rarely convenient. The pursuit of an ever-changing love object can be baffling, an obsession at once exhilarating and heartbreaking. The prize is never conquered, and an even more elaborate seduction might be required at the next turn. In the end, pursuit, not capture, is the true adventure.

In the twenty-first century, the metaphor of medicine as mistress is excessive. The singular male pursuit of a mistress is a nineteenth-century anachronism. Equal numbers of bright and dedicated young women now enter medicine, so the love object needs a sex change. We now also concede that loving partners might be of the same sex. Much has changed, and the innocence, some would say hypocrisy, of the mid-twentieth century is long gone. But, now, we can call doctors "providers," and patients, "customers" or "clients." I object to these words, which aim to cheapen the value of doctors and patients. Patients are sick people who come to see someone, hopefully, a doctor, who can, whether they might be cured or not, offer succor. We should not be in the business of running "product lines" to make widgets either. There are many diseases that can be cured and many that cannot, and sooner or later, all of us will die. The Aescalapion on the Isle of Cos was a holy place and still is. I have drunk from the waters of the well there and took, once again, the Hippocratic Oath in the temple on that island. Some powerful god or goddess still lives there. I cannot believe that "pathways" or "algorithms" in the hands of the uneducated can accomplish healing. Pursuit of a goddess using cookbook formulae is a masturbatory illusion. Given current approaches to the commercialization of medicine, I worry about the future of the care of the sick. Some of our students do not have the discipline or the skills required to elicit a complaint, obtain a careful history and perform an accurate physical examination. Processing whole populations through CAT or Magnetic Resonance Scanners could be simpler and even more revealing than rote untutored examinations. Such scans are advertised in newspapers and offered at a price. We possibly need a combination of both strategies: individual attention along with widget approaches to systems management. Given past efforts at Ford Motor Company and McNamara's performance during the Vietnam era, I worry about systems management for medicine.

Some "providers" prefer algorithms and guidelines. These may suffice, to some degree, in dealing with a single disease, but I remain, at heart, old school. Older patients usually have multiple disorders. I am attracted to a complicated and glamorous mistress, ever changing, demanding and, at times, exasperating. There remains in the art of medicine an eternal quality that will survive philistine assault. A siege upon a serious illness is much more complicated than can be depicted in a stick diagram. I guess Dr. Farber would have ordered a CAT scan for my sophomoric headache if one had been available. Later in life, when I became seriously ill due to infection following a ruptured appendix, I flew across the country to consult one of my own classmates who, on short notice, fit me into his busy Christmas Eve schedule.He took over an hour to obtain my history and complete the physical examination. He took blood pressures himself, and then walked with me to radiology to review a sheaf of useless CAT scans and Magnetic Resonance Arteriograms, ordered by others elsewhere. His approach was exactly what I had been taught and his care and concern saved my life.

Deans now combine a Master's in Business Administration with their medical degree. as qualifications for leadership. Money to be obtained from faculty who are supposed to teach, practice, and advance knowledge, has become the primary preoccupation of deanly endeavor. Pursuit of profit seems hardly adequate to inspire the passion that Dean McKewen told us about on our first shining day of medical school. Money, alone, cannot win a true and glamorous love. Devotion, passion, and attentiveness count for more. Tasteful and expensive gifts might help; the cost of our modern technology is so high that a touch of whoredom becomes inevitable. I hope we can come to terms with the expense of our new tools. I know, with their intelligent use, that we can do much better now than we did then. Those glorious days in medicine, when everything seemed new and possible, might once again be relived. I glimpse, from time to time, in students' eyes, ardor and true passion. And again, everything seems to be new and wondrous and possible.

WHAT I DID ON MY VACATION

Why do you seek rest, you were born to labor.
Thomas à Kempis

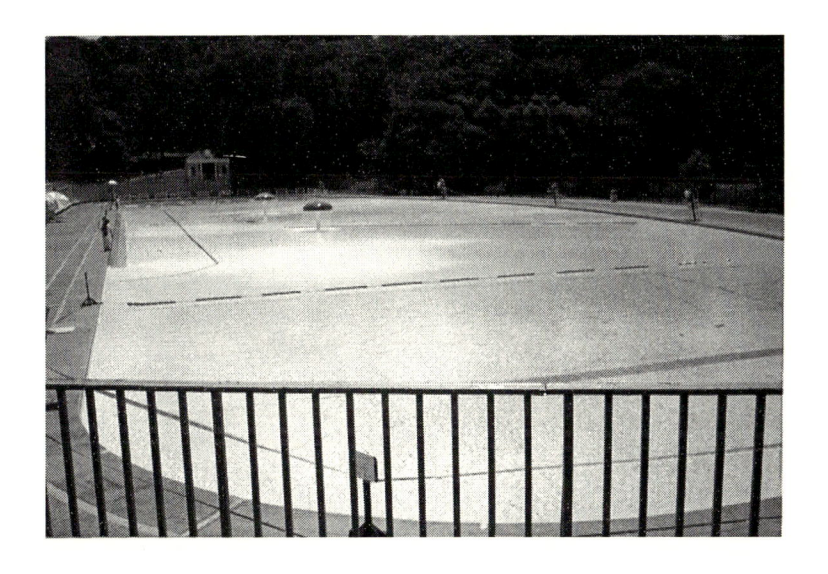

Tibbets Brook Park Pool

When I was ten years old, my father took me up Mount Vernon Avenue on top of the hill to buy me a used bicycle. I was a small kid and this was a 26-inch bicycle. I could barely stand up on it. So I would place one foot on the pedal and push with the other to get the bicycle rolling fast, then swing my other leg over. I also purchased a few tools at the bicycle store and learned to take care of the "wheel," as my father called it. I saved enough money from mowing lawns to buy a wicker basket for the handlebars.

Later that year, in November, my father died and we were suddenly very poor. The next summer vacation, I got a job working for "Doc" Wassermann, an old-fashioned druggist who had a small pharmacy at the foot of the hill in Sherwood Park. I sat in the back of the store on a stool in the corner, and watched him compound mystical medicament with mortar and pestle, following doctors' instructions written in Latin flourishes on prescriptions. Then I would take my bicycle and ride around Sherwood Park in Yonkers and the eastern part of Mount Vernon to deliver his hand-mixed medicines.

Doc Wassermann, a small, tidy man with a brush mustache, always wore a spotless shirt and a bow tie. He was quiet and kind and paid me four dollars a week. Those four dollars a week were important to me. Just after my father died, I took cornet lessons to play in the school band, but my mother could not afford the four dollars to buy that instrument. So, four dollars a week, symbolically, meant a great deal. I worked until the drugstore closed at about nine o'clock and then delivered medicines to patients' homes in the late evening. The little wicker basket in the front of the bicycle held precious cargo, and I happily sped up and down the hills of the Sherwood Park. I had once seen a statue of Mercury with winged feet: I pretended to be like him. With each delivery were warm welcomes and a small tip when I got to my destinations, which were usually modest little homes.

Doc Wassermann also treated people who just came in to the store for advice. He seemed to know exactly what kind of cough medicine to dispense and did so quietly and efficiently. Later in life, when I was fifteen, I developed an unpleasant and annoying complaint, anal pruritis. This seemed to come about after I had done a great deal of swimming in heavily chlorinated pools. This condition was absolutely agonizing and also embarrassing, there is nothing worse than being seen scratching your rear end in public. I went down to the Bronx to see Dr. Gerard Carroll. He examined the area and quickly wrote a prescription that I took to Wassermann's pharmacy. The kindly druggist continued to fill my prescription, a tan granular ointment dispensed in a small thick jar. This was absolutely specific in relieving my annoying problem. I used this treatment for years, even after Dr. Carroll died. Finally, Doc Wassermann closed his store, and I could no longer get the precious unction. I still wish I knew what was in it. The only substitute was cortisone, which was not nearly as effective.

Wassermann's pharmacy did not have a soda fountain. I spent some of my earnings to buy ice cream sodas and treated my friends to ice cream sundaes and banana splits; the rest, I put in a bank account. On Doc Wassermann's recommendation, I later got a job over on Riverdale Avenue, near the Hudson River, as a "soda jerk" at another drug store. By then, I was twelve, an age when this was an important and popular job. I learned to mix cherry cokes, chocolate floats, malteds and all the delicious things that old-fashioned soda fountains dispensed in those days. My friends would come all the way over to Riverdale Avenue just to have me mix special sodas. I had to wear a little white hat and took some kidding about that, but there was also a benefit. I could have whatever I wanted to eat or drink.

Still, there was not much money for me in this kind of work. So by the time I was thirteen, my friends and I began to caddie on weekends. We worked at Sprain Lake and at Grassy Sprain public golf courses and country clubs in Scarsdale. We received $1.50 a bag and $3.00 for doubles. The best place to caddie was Sprain Lake, which was called a "semiprivate" course because Westchester County ran it. Periodically, Joe Lewis would come to play amidst a great entourage of noisy hangers-on. I could tell that he was uncomfortable playing with these noisy people when I caddied for this group and actually spoke with the "Brown Bomber." He was a reticent man but he, somehow, conveyed that he felt badly that he had to come with this entourage, many of whom were white, but it was the only way he could get on a course to play golf.

I had a talk with the pro at Sprain Lake about Mr. Lewis'

problem. He told me that if Mr. Lewis and I would like to come early to do a singleton, he would let us tee off at about 6:00 a.m. So, all that summer when I was thirteen years old, I would wait for Joe Lewis on Central Avenue in Yonkers at dawn. He drove a 1947 Chevrolet sedan and he always had fruit on the front seat. He would pick me up at Central Avenue, we would drive North to Tuckahoe Road, and then to Sprain Lake and promptly tee off at six in the morning. The course was always deserted. Mr. Lewis could hit the ball a consistently good 270 yards down the middle of the fairway. He never talked much, we never lost any balls, and his shots never landed in the rough. He was not much interested in approach shots or putting and was a little bit impatient there, but he was a superb athlete. It was an honor to caddie for him. After our round, he would pay $3 for the singleton. His canvass golf bag was quite light and three dollars was the usual fee, with tip, for carrying two heavy leather bags owned by duffers and stuffed with clubs. We were usually done in two hours. So, by 8:30 in the morning, he took a detour to drop me off at my home on Kimball Avenue. The boys in the neighborhood would all sit perched on my stop, waiting for our appearance. Mr. Lewis would wave to them through the car window. They believed that I was getting boxing tips from the champ: I continued to let them believe this fiction. Actually, he and I rarely talked at all. He would offer me a peach or a pear, one before we went on the course and one, after the round. In spite of the avuncular relationship, I came to feel close to him.

During the wintertime, by the time I was thirteen, I began to work at pin setting in a bowling alley in downtown Yonkers. The boss insisted that we get Social Security cards and I had to be at least fourteen, or older. So I inflated my age by two years, using my confirmation name, Ralph Francis. This act, five decades later, caused innumerable bureaucratic complications. After paying Social Security deductions for more than half a century, the agency notified me that I was non-existent. Many years later, a patient of mine who worked at the CIA in Langley had requested my curriculum vitae for a possible position. They called back several times to get my Social Security number and when they got it, the agent who had offered me a position notified me about "an irregularity." While I was really not interested in working for "the company," I was interested in clearing my Social Security record. I went to the main office in Fairfax, Virginia, with my birth certificate to straighten out my youthful deception. The clerks there were polite and helpful; apparently, this was not an uncommon occurrence. I have just started to get payments for those years of labor.

Pin setting was dangerous work. Perched on a partition between pits, we manned two alleys on busy nights. After the first shot, we quickly leapt into each pit after the first ball rolled down to clear the area for the spare shot. After the second roll, we pushed a foot lever that caused fine guides to protrude to set pins by hand, juggling two in each hand and placing one onto each spot. Later, overhead racks became available. It was dark and dusty back there, and you had to leap back and forth quickly to be sure the spare ball didn't run you down. On occasion, the bowlers, drunk or vicious, and sometimes both, would actually try to nail pin boys. This happened a couple of times to my fiery Sicilian friend, Vinnie Tuccino. He crawled out from beneath the façade, stood in the alley and rolled a ball right back at the offending group. He followed up by running up the alley, confronting four frightened men with raised fists. The manager threw the unruly group out and put Vinnie right back to work.

The money was good, but the hours were late, and the back of the alley was dark and dusty. A massive three-hundred pound professional named Bill Gruner, who had rolled many perfect games, ran one of the places on McLean Avenue where we worked. Bill got Vinnie (as soon as he was old enough to) and me, to go around collecting money from scattered vending and gaming machines and jukeboxes in the Bronx. He liked and trusted us, so we drove his big Packard sedan for this task. After a while, he suggested that, since we were collecting a good bit of money and there was some competition, we probably should carry guns. He actually offered to give us each a small handgun. It was quite obvious where this job would have taken us. Had we followed this path, our lives would have been radically different. The money was good and we were sorely tempted.

By then, I was swimming competitively, and luckily, decided to get out of the pin setting and collecting business. I, then, began to work for the YMCA because my swimming coach, Mr. David Smith, was the physical director there. He saw to it that I practiced regularly, so during the summers when I was fifteen and sixteen years old, I worked as a counselor for the YMCA day camp. One of the things counselors had to do was control a group of nine and ten-year-old boys. I also had to lead a prayer every morning. Dave left it up to me to figure out what prayer to say. So, the night before, I would stop by the Christian Science Reading Room to copy the latest prayer in the *Christian Science Monitor*. The next morning, I would recite this absolutely spectacular prayer. Mr. Smith was always curious about where I got these inspiring masterpieces. I never actually lied, but he believed that I was making them up.

The worse thing that could happen to the YMCA day camp was to have a rainy day. Then, we showed movies using an old 16mm projector. One particular reel showed Africans actually being eaten by alligators. The film was real. You could see an arm and a leg coming off here and there and people frantically trying to get out of the bloody water. I would show this film on rainy mornings, but if the boys were at all disruptive, the threat to withhold the showing never failed to keep them in line. The bloodthirsty boys never tired of watching the alligators eat the Africans. There were, however, some funny things about the YMCA. The creepy little male general secretary would hide in the locker room and peer through the cracks in the locker to see what was going on. I guess his hope was to catch someone jacking off. The coach, when we told him about this, made him stop.

During the winter of my senior year in high school, I worked in a well-equipped physics laboratory at Alexander Smith's and Sons carpet factory in the Nepperhan Valley. That fine opportunity came about because I scored highly on a citywide aptitude test in mathematics and physics. I was assigned to work in the research physics laboratory. The head of the laboratory sat at a desk, stationed exactly in the middle of the large room. He spent all of his time reading technical magazines. He was delighted when I repaired a huge hand-cranked static electricity machine that I found in a dusty closet. When wound up, it generated a loud crack and spark. Connection of the hand crank to a spare electric motor yielded even more power. The director had me crank up this gadget whenever visitors came to the laboratory. The Frankenstein appearance and the continual loud snapping of forty thousand-volt electric sparks never failed to impress visiting executives. Of course, this spectacular display was absolutely useless. I kept busy doing useful things like making sure that carpet dye lots were similar on a day-to-day basis, using a spectrophotometer and measuring the physical characteristics of various types of synthetic and wool fibers. To help with these measurements, Dr. Paul Agron, a curiously sad former atomic researcher at Argon National Laboratory, taught me differential and integral calculus in my senior year of high school. I was not to understand his sadness until later in my life when, as an air force officer with a Top Secret clearance, I visited a facility in Las Vegas and saw row upon row of hydrogen bombs.

In 1948, Harry Truman ran for president against Thomas Dewey. Mr. Truman came in late summer to campaign at the steamy factory in the valley. I stood right next to this energetic man with his wire spectacles and gleaming blue eyes. He spoke honestly and fervently to the workers gathered in the factory yard. He clearly understood what they faced in their day-to-day labors and what it meant to be a workingman. It was no surprise that he defeated the stodgy Dewey hands down in the election in the fall.

By that time, I was able to support my first car, a beautiful 1933 Plymouth Coupe. I commuted from Kimball Avenue to Roosevelt High School, then to Smith's carpet factory and then on to the YMCA to practice swimming by five in the afternoon. By the time I was seventeen, I got to be a lifeguard at Tibbetts Brook Park. This was a huge swimming pool in Yonkers near the Bronx border. The pool was 140 yards long and about 50 yards wide at its middle. There were two deeper ends, each about 33 yards wide. Five lifeguards were always on duty. We had a lot fun but also worked hard at Tibbetts Brook. The head of the lifeguards was a tall basketball star named Bob Christopher. Bob and I were good friends, but he never thought much of swimmers. He thought that anyone who was a good swimmer just had to practice for a long time and needed little talent.

A tall, lanky, dark-haired policeman named "Spider" patrolled the outside of the pool. He would lean over the parapet and call out things like, "What week is this?" There would come a chorus from below, "It's national cherry week." He would say, "What about it?" and then the chorus would reply, "Everyone's gotta get one." The girls would giggle and cover up their laughter. During the weekends, gangs of tough guys came up from New York City. After we got off watch on our chairs, each lifeguard would have to walk around the pool perimeter carrying a stick and looking tough. This was called the guinea stick, because most of the troublemakers were Italians. We were supposed to stick our chests out and flex our muscles to make sure that peace was kept. We averaged fifteen of sixteen pullouts or rescues during weekends, when the pool was crowded.

One Saturday, a tall good-looking girl attempted a back flip off the diving board, striking her head on the end of the board. I could see immediately that she was unconscious as she slowly sank to the twelve-foot depth. I was manning the middle chair in the deep end. I jumped from the chair to the end of the board she had just left, got a good spring and retrieved her within seconds. She was unconscious when I put her over my back in the "fireman's carry" and started running to the lifeguard station. She woke up to find herself draped over my back. For some inexplicable reason, she promptly bonded and fell in love with me. This was a tall girl. She was 6'2", six inches taller than I. She became quite devoted to me. She would wait for me to get off the chair and accompany me on my round-the-pool police walks. I felt the object of unspoken ridicule and repeatedly pled with her not to accompany me during this patrol. She towered over me, emphasizing my stature, making me a less-credible authority figure in spite of my guinea stick. We met secretly and I never dated her because I was too self-conscious or, really, too insecure. Instead, we went out parking in her car. She was a fine young woman and a talented artist. I saw that she had made drawings of me, which were shown here and there in town. I know now that I hurt her with this shabby treatment, but what could be expected from a silly adolescent who worried about a disparity in height?

We, lifeguards, threw terrific parties, and there was never a shortage of girls who attended. Whenever a friendly police officer was on duty, we would sneak into the pool with girlfriends in the dark of night to swim. One of the guards, Howie, had a peculiar trick. He was able to emerge from the bottom of the 12-foot depth with just his rear end sticking out. He had an unusually hairy butt. There were floodlights at the deep end, which were usually kept darkened. We asked the girls if they would like to see the moon over Tibbetts. Howie would then slip into the water at the shallows and quietly swim under water to the deep end. The spotlights would be turned on and this odd animal-looking object would surface, remain for a minute, and then mysteriously submerge. The lights then went out. It was hard to tell exactly what the object was, but slowly, it would dawn on the girls that it was a huge, hairy rear end. But no one could tell whose it was because we all got in the water at the same time.

When I was accepted to medical school, I needed more money. So I went to work as a laborer. At this time, I had a friend, a short burly sidekick named Johnny Fokine. Johnny was in engineering school, and he was perfectly happy to work where I did and go along with me. He was shy and reticent, but quite bright and we became good friends, although as with Joe Lewis and I, we never talked much at all. In the summer of my junior year in college, we got a job stacking cinder blocks in a factory that manufactured them. We had to stack the blocks in such a way that the forklifts could pick them up and load them for transport. The brick factory was on the banks of the Hudson River and it was a steaming hot summer. The steam coming from the plant and the humidity and heat, made for almost inhuman working conditions. There was no shade. It was like a scene out of hell.

The work seemed deceptively easy at first, and I paired up with a small wiry African American. We entered into a good-natured competition, and for every block he stacked, I stacked one, too. About 10:00 in the morning, instead of 6-inch blocks, they brought out the "ball busters." All the workers groaned, because these were the 12-inch blocks. About the time the "ball busters" came out, we had a break. My partner offered to buy me a beer. We both gulped our beers quickly and, again, started to match stacking, block for block. Suddenly, I experienced painful and uncontrollable spasms in my hand and arms. Then, both my upper limbs spastically curled up into my chest. My partner said, "Man, the boss sees you, we lose this job." I had gotten employment through the International Hod Carriers and Laborers Union. He and the union steward hid me in some shade under a storage shed by the river, feeding me salt tablets and water. I recovered enough to work in the afternoon. That was a terrible job, but Johnny was a lot smarter than I was. He did not try to match anyone block for block. I learned another lesson here. We had a sort of truck that gathered us up in the morning and we regularly picked up a Polish workingman from Nodine Hill. The poor soul had been ordered to this work by a judge to pay his overdue alimony. This seemed to me to be like a sentence to hell, a terrible punishment, and an important lesson to learn about marital misjudgments. The poor guy had a dream. His dream, about which he constantly ruminated, was a job with the Nash Fence Company. I never found out whether or not he escaped from the cinder block sentence.

Luckily, the Westchester Park Commission was looking for

lifeguards and they remembered me from Tibbetts Brook. I coached Johnny in rescue techniques and we worked the rest of that summer at Rye Beach and Pool on Long Island Sound. This was an interesting place to work because the lifeguards covered both the beach and the pool. Rye Beach was great. We swam laps in the pool and rotated watches between the pool and the sound. We had a little rowboat in the sound, and the pace was not as frantic as it was at Tibbetts. The clientele was much more refined than the toughs at Tibbets, and two large lady lifeguards worked there as well. They enjoyed wrestling, boat races, and jokes, and were generally agreeable, rounding out a pleasant group of young people.

A favorite early morning task consisted of raking up the seaweed from the beach and loading the smelly stuff into a real dump truck. We then got to operate this great truck to dump seaweed into a remote corner of the park. We competed to get the chance to drive the truck. Usually, I got to do this with a burly weight lifter. The boss seemed to like our enthusiasm and the girls were not at all interested in this task. The truck had a sputtery motor and when we finished dumping seaweed, we had to park it in a garage. We stopped for breakfast in the amusement park, then walked back to our stations. One morning, just as we parked the truck, the engine caught fire in the garage and would not start. We looked around frantically for an extinguisher. Fuel and other trucks were nestled close by in that dark garage. Not knowing what else to do, we opened the hood, stood up on the radiator, and both peed on the engine. Our prompt action put out the fire. We were lucky to be young and to have unimpeded flow, and it was also fortunate that the girls were not driving the truck. The smell was not good and our boss was pretty unhappy with us. After that, we were not permitted drive the truck anymore. Our enthusiasm for raking and shoveling seaweed waned considerably.

As at Tibbets, the other good things about the lifeguard job were girls and late-night parties on a real beach. We could get on free rides at Playland and our social life was lively. I became particularly attracted to a well-endowed brown-eyed girl in a two-piece, leopard-skin bathing suit. The minute I saw her climbing out of the pool, checking her barely contained and ample breasts carefully, I realized that she was someone I needed to know much better. I did more than "lust in my heart" and we began dating on Fridays and Sundays. On Saturday night, the serious date night, I drove out to New Jersey to see a petite, blonde blue-eyed graduate student. One Saturday morning, I woke up and looked into the big brown eyes of the leopard-bathing suit girl. Between those placid eyes and breasts with areolae the size of silver dollars, the image of a cow floated involuntarily into my mind. She was a nice girl, but try as I might, I was unable to erase the bovine image.

This disrespectful and capricious thought failed to do justice to a gentle girl from a good family. A skilled stenographer and typist, she helped me compose a report for my cardiac clinic rotation at Lenox Hill Hospital that summer. In matters such as this, the heart is cruel and idiosyncratic. This random thought, that summer vacation, determined the choice of my life's partner and the genes of our four fine children. The petite blond from New Jersey and I eventually married.

I needed still more support to afford medical school and a friend of mine made a contact for me with the International Brotherhood of Teamsters. I got a job in steel lathing, the rebars that are used to reinforce concrete. This was basically an Irish union but some Italians were also members. Johnny and I carried steel lathing for the concrete forms, for the columns of a bridge that was being built over the Hutchinson Parkway. The job paid six dollars an hour, an enormous sum in those times. We got up early in the morning and worked until three in the afternoon. During the first week, we were absolutely exhausted, suffering sore backs and forearms. We wondered how our fellow workers could play softball at the end of the day.

Johnny and I gradually got the knack of it and our backs got stronger. We then began to compete to see how much steel we could move. We could move a lot of steel in a short amount of time. Finally, a union boss came over to us saying, "Hey, boys, what are you going to do in September?" We told him we were going back to school. He smiled gently and said, "You see these guys? Some of them are forty years old and they got to keep doing this for the rest of their lives. Slow up." We slowed up. I had developed great respect for these workingmen because most had served in World War II. At lunch, they compared notes about the best way to take out a German tank, including the most effective way to derail treads, when to throw a grenade, and how to shoot the enemy emerging from the hatches. There was no doubt that these capable and brave men actually had done these things. I, still, am proud of my two union cards, the Hod Carriers and the Teamsters, and I keep them in an old wallet in my bureau drawer.

I also worked during Easter and Christmas vacations. For two Easter vacations, while in college, I worked at A.S. Beck Shoes downtown on 14th Street in Manhattan. They initially hired me as a wrapper, but I was not a good wrapper. None of the ladies liked the way I wrapped their shoeboxes. To this day, I still do not wrap packages. I always buy gifts, whenever possible, in shops that do wrapping. So, they put me out on the floor selling shoes. These were cheap shoes and if the ladies complained of the fit, which many did, I had to take the shoes back to the manager, Mr. Shapiro, a tall, bald man who brandished a shoe stretcher. He would stand up, place a shoe on the last, holding this tool and the shoe high in the air while twisting the handle vigorously. He then sent me to refit the shoes again with instructions to "rub their ankles and feet bit." I was then a skinny good-looking kid with a lot of hair. The women always thought the shoes felt better the second time I put them on. But I came to find out that the shoe stretcher really did not stretch shoes at all. The rotating screw was stripped completely. These cheap shoes would have come apart had the stretcher actually worked. A hit as a salesman, Mr. Shapiro wanted me to continue working there. He thought I had a future in selling shoes. His enthusiasm was flattering, but that was the only thing good about that job.

Christmas came and I still needed money, so in the height of the Christmas rush, I went to work at Macy's on Herald Square. The store gave us an elaborate course on how to fill out various charge slips: Macy's charge, C.O.D., other credit cards, and finally, cash and carry. These were very complex forms. It took a week to learn how to fill them out and they had to be done in quadruplicate, with various carbons going here and there. I never really learned to complete these forms. I got my customers to pay cash and take their purchases home, telling them that this would be far safer. The gift shop where I was assigned, again, catered mainly to ladies. I knew nothing about the inventory and every now and then, customers would come in asking for "a lazy Susan" or a "trivet." Initially, I had no idea what these things were but I quickly learned. I would walk around the counters trying to be charming until the lady found what she wanted. I never completed any of the complicated Macy's charges, charge sent or C.O.D. slips. This position, during the Christmas rush, was hard work—much harder, in some ways, than working as a laborer. Some overbearing floorwalker was always watching how many times you went to the bathroom, or for a smoke, and you could not, ever, sit down. I felt sorry for the clerks who had to do this work the rest of their lives. However, many seemed to enjoy it. The eagle eye out for the number of times you went to the bathroom was particularly offensive to me. I still go out of my way to be especially nice to sales people in department stores.

By the summer of my senior year in medical school, I did something that related to medicine; I got a position with the Schering Drug Company detailing doctors in the offices on Park and Fifth Avenues. Prednisone had just become available. I learned all about Prednisone and visited doctors on behalf of the Schering Corporation. My cachet as a medical student was supposed to get me into the offices for a required number of detailing visits per day. I carried an inventory of samples in the trunk of my car parked in midtown Manhattan, changing to the other side of the street in mid-morning to accommodate daily parking rules. Getting past receptionists was tough, but when I told them I was a medical student, I usually saw the doctor himself. This was really an unfair advantage. To this day, anytime detail people come to my office, they are immediately accommodated so they can put me down as a call. I insist that they do this no matter how brief or perfunctory our interactions. Detailing was my last vacation job. So, this is what I did on my vacations. I worked. I still work on vacations that are often arranged around medical meetings. Remembering those past jobs, I am grateful I have a profession that I love so much. I find it hard to stop working. Whenever I see a working person with an illness or injury, I am as liberal as I can be to grant time for their recovery. Almost all of them want to work. Few working people get up in the morning planning to do a bad job. They all deserve respect and understanding. My union cards reside safely in an old worn wallet in the top dresser drawer.

SEVILLENAS: AN AUDITION

Dicebamus hesterna die—as we were saying yesterday.
Luis de Leon, on resuming lectures at Salamanca after
four years of inquisition.

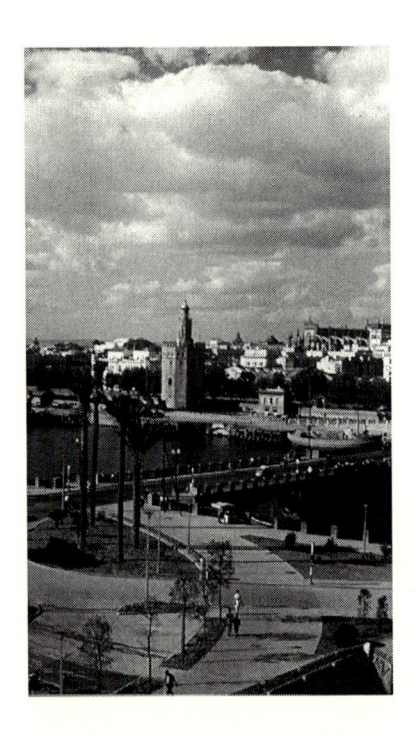

View from Calle Asuncion, Seville, Spain

Moron de la Frontera seemed to be a million miles from the Bronx, particularly after a two-day journey by a military transport propeller craft from New York to Madrid, then, on a C47 to the base in southern Spain. The tarmac at the Strategic Air Command runway, thirty-five miles from the city of Seville, shimmered in the glaring August heat. Colonel Tom Lomax Morgan, the hospital commander, was waiting to meet me. A quiet, shy West Texan and former general practitioner, he had joined the air force after his divorce, and was now, judging by his wings, a senior flight surgeon. In spite of my protests, he picked up my heavy suitcase insisting on lugging it himself to the staff car. He drove me to the Bachelor Officers' Quarters where I was to reside as an unaccompanied officer.

I had sought this assignment in Spain after winding down my second year of surgical residency with a pathology rotation at St. Luke's Hospital in New York City. With a draft obligation for military service as a doctor, Spain seemed an exciting choice. I had read about the new Strategic Air Command bases in the *New York Times* and was intrigued. I had never been to Europe or traveled abroad and, after a trip to Washington and a claim of Spanish fluency, I received orders to report to this exciting post in Andalucia.

To join me for a two-year tour, my wife would have to pay her way. But she would, I was assured, be welcome. Eve had decided to remain behind for six months after my departure to continue working in the Department of Anatomy at New York University. As Colonel Morgan and I sat side by side in a blue Ford staff car, he chewed on his worn pipe anxiously, which, I soon learned, was a characteristic gesture. He spoke hesitantly. "You are the new surgeon?" He asked almost apologetically, "Can you deliver babies?" "Well, I delivered them as a medical student, but I have been a surgical resident." "Well, do you think you can do obstetrics?" I said, "Probably, if I review a bit."

The colonel went on, in his quiet, halting manner, to describe a near panic among expectant mothers on the base. Two women had died in childbirth, one of them the wife of the previous chief of obstetrics and gynecology. She had suffered a fat embolism during delivery under spinal anesthesia. Colonel Morgan asked me to deliver babies under local anesthesia, if at all possible. He seemed relieved when I agreed to this. Fortunately, all my new textbooks had been shipped in a footlocker. This was lucky for me, as we had no library. I had purchased the best current textbooks of medicine, pediatrics, obstetrics and gynecology as well as psychiatry and neurology. The trunk contained all three surgical texts and two books on orthopedics, including closed reduction of fractures. The books on obstetrics and fractures were to prove initially most critical.

Several good Spanish obstetricians practiced in Seville, so I apprenticed myself, informally, to one of them. From him, I learned the practice of the Read method of natural childbirth with minimal analgesia. His motto was, "If you give it to the mother, you give it to the baby." The technique involved careful pre-delivery instruction, something practiced widely now but done rarely in obstetrical practice at that time. Part of my duties was to attend to patients in downtown Seville in a hospital the air force had rented from a local surgeon. The five-story building was called "El Cano," and it was a pretty place, flanked by palm and lemon trees with peacocks strutting in its well-tended gardens. The Spanish obstetrician was a good teacher; I regained confidence in handling routine deliveries. I reviewed over and over the lessons of my clerkship in OB/GYN to be sure I knew why and when forceps were indicated. The first time I needed forceps, the nurse queried, "What kind?" "Classic," was my reply since I had read that these were the safest. Actually, forceps application should be rare since these tricky instruments can cause cerebral palsy due to head injury. To this day, I respect the challenges of obstetric practice. Most deliveries are easy, however, the complications of childbirth tax even the most skilled surgeons. I thought about my own delivery at home in the Bronx by our general practitioner, Dr. Gerald Carroll.

Compared to surgery, obstetrics was fun, and in many ways, a happier specialty. I encouraged husbands to be present in the delivery room, something rarely done in 1958. A master sergeant, married to a vivacious French lady, had enthusiastically attended the prenatal instructions with his wife. However, at the last moment, the husband lost his nerve and did not want to be in the room. During second stage labor, as the head crowned, the woman began joking and laughing loudly. The burly sergeant abruptly stuck his head into the room, unmasked and ungowned. I said, "You are welcome in here, but you have to put on a mask." He demanded angrily, "What is going on here? She only laughs like that when she has sex." Rarely, and in spite of inevitable pain, childbirth might be a pleasurable or possibly, a sexual experience. This was the only time I observed this, however.

Obstetrical events were not always uneventful in that environment. One night, our fine chief nurse summoned me from the officers' quarters with great urgency. A senior diplomat's wife was in delivery and in major distress. I questioned her carefully inasmuch as there was a Spanish obstetrician in attendance. This nurse from Austin, Texas replied in a broad drawl, "For Chrissakes Raff, just come." I sped thirty miles from base to El Cano to find a ragged perineal tear being repaired such that the major lip was being sewn to the minor lip. The result was totally unacceptable in appearance. Tapping a slender and sweaty fellow on the shoulder—this was the first time I had seen him—I said, "Move over." After anesthetizing the perineum, I then removed every last crude catgut suture in order to start over. The unfortunate lady was agitated and had been, I was told, screaming loudly from the start. After intravenous sedation, the ragged wound was carefully sutured while the erstwhile obstetric surgeon hung over my shoulder, muttering. His mask dangled below a haughty Spanish nose.

The next morning, Colonel Morgan was uncharacteristically disturbed. He worried that I had created an "international incident." I had asked this surgeon about his OB/GYN training. He informed me proudly that he had "gone to Vienna to observe." Furthermore, the mask was worn below the nose because no pathogens lived in the nasal passages. I told him, "Well, that is not good enough. You had better actually learn something about obstetrics." Tact, unfortunately, was never my strong point, particularly in dealing with poor patient care. In all fairness, this surgeon, as did all European medical students, had simply read to pass examinations in the clinical specialties. They were not required, as were American and British students, to attend as clinical clerks and obtain hands-on experience.

We covered two separate facilities, the El Cano Clinic in Seville for dependents, and the Moron de la Frontera Air Base, and considerable tension existed among the professional staff.

Thirty-five miles was a safe distance for an atomic blast in the opinion of Generalismo Franco. The airfield was, therefore, situated at that distance from the city of Seville. Unfortunately, we were staffed as a single unit because of bureaucratic oversight. We cared for aircrews and ground support for six SAC B-47 bombers stationed at the base, a tactical air command squadron, and a few dependants in base housing. Most of the families lived in Seville. With a complement of six doctors, we slept in about every third night at each site. The air force also employed two Spanish contract physicians. I had reservations about the capabilities of these physicians as well as about their discipline. They were pleasant enough under ordinary circumstances, but their almost total lack of concern and fatalism about complications was disturbing.

A slender, attractive young woman appeared late one afternoon at El Cano emergency room complaining of abdominal pain and vaginal spotting. She had missed her last period. In spite of a falling hematocrit and physical findings, which should have suggested an ectopic pregnancy, she had been sent home twice from the emergency room in Seville. The third time she reappeared, I was asked to come in from the airbase to examine her.

I did her third pelvic examination, detecting a tender mass to the right of the uterus. I told the contract surgeon that she had an ectopic pregnancy and scheduled her for surgery. He was reluctant to agree to this diagnosis. We found a bleeding tubal pregnancy, and I was quite direct in pointing this out to him. Even after the ruptured swollen uterine appendage was placed in a jar, he shook his head mournfully, denying the obvious diagnosis. An ability for self-deception is one of the most dangerous pitfalls in patient care. I believe that self-delusion and poor medicine go hand in hand. I grew to appreciate more and more the strict discipline and long hours that we, American medical students and residents, had endured.

In spite of what many would consider a desirable assignment, some Americans, mainly wives, stationed in Spain, hated the place. They adapted poorly to the foreign culture. Initially, no base housing existed and few Spaniards spoke English. Distraught women in hair curlers appeared at sick call. "I hate Spain!" was recorded over and over as a chief complaint. Sometimes, charts read: CC "hates Spain," RX "home on next available transport." Sometimes, this had to be done for several reasons. Some wives, with limited education, could not adjust to living abroad. They could not speak the language nor appreciate the culture. Sometimes, their husbands would either be sleeping with an elegant Spanish lady or having an affair with the maid. Air force personnel were paid, by Spanish standards, enormous salaries. Full-time household help could be had for about $10.00 a month and all of early base support staff initially lived "on the economy." Average Americans did not adapt well to an expatriate lifestyle. Air force personnel were required to dress in civilian clothes, including coat and tie, in the town. The combination of "sargentos" with lots of money in their pockets and ambitious Spanish ladies was explosive. This cultural dissonance occurred wherever in Spain our military went, in spite of efforts to synthesize a "Little America" at each base including a post exchange, a motion picture theater with popcorn, and a fully staffed hospital. At the same time, the spectacle of all that wealth in the hands of relatively uncultured people corrupted the locals.

The wives' "cry wolf" complaints caused dangerous medical misunderstandings. Later, during my obstetrical experience, I changed shift on a Sunday morning with the same contract physician responsible for the missed ectopic. A woman was presented to me as she remained in prolonged labor. He described the case as, "Typical American wife, just not pushing and not working." "She has been in labor for how long"? I asked. "Oh, about eighteen hours," was the reply. Actually, at 10:00 A.M. that Sunday morning, she had been in labor for well over twenty-four hours. She was seriously dehydrated and exhausted. I performed the "classic" maneuvers of Leopold to determine fetal location. The baby was clearly in a transverse position and would have never delivered vaginally. This time, I coaxed my colleague a bit more diplomatically. He stayed to help with the Caesarean section, proving, this time, to be a willing and capable assistant.

All the doctors at the base were fulfilling military obligations required at that time. Our ages ranged from twenty-five to twenty-eight years old. Specialty interests were represented although none of us had finished a residency. We were all fledglings. With two years of experience, I was designated "chief of surgery," with a year of internship. Jimmy Craig from Tennessee, the youngest of the lot, was a pediatrician, as was Dr. Richard Ryan from Milwaukee. Alyosha Kendrick had a year of internal medicine and was aiming to practice this specialty. Later, a well-qualified genial southern gentleman from Georgia assumed all OB responsibilities but took no other call. This led to continual grumbling since we still needed to cover the two sites. But he did a fine job with obstetrics. We had to staff both a civilian and a military mission. For this reason, I later supported, and continue to support, our military medical school at the Uniformed Services University of the Health Sciences in Bethesda, Maryland. Compared to every other night during surgical residency, third-night call was a great luxury. The pay and the living conditions in Spain were a dramatic relief compared to our former poverty in New York. I learned fluent Spanish and could get along quite well on the economy. But my life was basically schizophrenic, divided between the airmen on the base and obligations in town. I stayed in the Bachelor Officers' Quarters, and got into town for deliveries, operations, and fracture reductions.

The air base at Moron de la Frontera was a fascinating place. The Strategic Air Command Squadron had six B-47 bombers, armed with hydrogen bombs and targeted at the Ukraine. The Cold War was at its height. These SAC officers were never allowed to drink alcohol. These air crews were on an immediate "reflex call." At the sound of a raucous klaxon, they would speed to the runway and sometimes start their engines. The latter was considered to be, and indeed was, a serious event. The Tactical Air Squadron men, between flight exercises, spent their spare time partying and drinking at the Officer's Club. I was privileged to serve with the

First Fighter Day Squadron commanded by Colonel Chuck Yeager. The SAC and TAC flyers, though temperamentally different, were some of the finest men I have ever met. I became a close friend of several fliers who became fans of the awe-aspiring bullfights in Seville. In my 1957 Chevrolet convertible, Lieutenant Don Holzman and I made a memorable trip to the wine harvest at Jerez de la Frontera. After a night of heavy wine intake, we stumbled to the bathroom. There sat a female whose task was to hand a grimy towel to its patrons. When we unzipped, she became frankly nosy in attempting to inspect American equipment. Her overt curiosity undid us both. Neither of us could relax enough to empty our brimming bladders. We tipped her a handful of pesetas, and blundered into some nearby thatch to relieve ourselves. Urinary inhibitions quickly faded as we saw that most Spanish men urinated freely on the side of the road. This act, a symbol of male independence, was convenient and probably healthy. I learned to urinate handily, eventually ignoring "los cuartos de baño" and the crones who attended them.

Fighter pilots, as might be expected, were aggressively adventuresome. Their main medical problems resulted from visits to "ventas," outdoor nightclubs, which featured beautiful flamenco dancers. Some of these girls also plied the oldest profession, but some did it for love. Male flamenco dancers were generally gay. The pilots' usual complaints were urinary. Slight burning, minor discharge or urgency would lead to immediate sick call at the dispensary. The original flight surgeon was a rigid Hispanic Catholic. He was unpopular because he sternly lectured the men. This approach caused both embarrassment and hostility and was counterproductive since some of the men would not report to sick call. I took a liberal Bronx attitude: after getting cultures and a urinalysis, I usually prescribed a combination of penicillin and bicillin or an appropriate antibiotic. The sympathetic approach attracted the loyalty of the fighter contingent. I made an effort to find out all about the antibiotic sensitivities of *gonococcus* in the fly zone of our F-100s. I, then, concocted a mixture of potent oral antibiotics to be taken before and immediately after exposure. In those days before HIV, the approach appeared safe and effective. But I would not now recommend such an approach. The large capsules became known as Doc DePalma's "no-sweat pills."

As I was about the same age as my flying friends, I became less lonely. We played poker in the BOQ and traveled to towns in Andalusia, went to bullfights and flamenco parties in the Ventas. I once remarked to Colonel Yeager that I would never leave New York City. "Well, you had better go have a steak in Kansas City," he replied. We eventually did just that when we got back to the United States. I later left New York to discover the fine people who populated the rest of the United States.

A tragic automobile accident crippled the assigned flight surgeon, so I was elected temporary flight surgeon without portfolio. Colonel Morgan oversaw my work. As I began giving more medical care to these officers, I was told that I should go flying with them. Colonel Yeager was never much for regulations. Although I had never been checked through the altitude chamber, I became an eager passenger in the TAC fighters. I learned to maneuver from the back seat of an F100-F; barrel rolls were my specialty. The fighter jocks were delighted inasmuch as the former flight surgeon had taken his four-hour monthly flight time requirements in a sedate C47 transport called a "Gooney Bird." Colonel Morgan convinced me that I should stay an extra year in Spain so that I could attend the School of Aviation Medicine in San Antonio. I became interested in aviation medicine and flying, both of which caused me to reappraise my career goals. The drudgery of junior surgical residency did not, at first glance, compare at all with this glamorous life.

The combination of beautiful Spanish women, warm nights, flamenco dancing, and young airmen led to explosive and epidemic venereal disease. Gonorrhea was rampant and syphilis itself was not uncommon in southern Spain. African American airmen were welcomed by the local ladies and they enjoyed those equal opportunities. Since many of the non-commissioned officers were rednecks, whenever an airman, particularly an African American, developed venereal disease, the offender was detailed to lawn mowing in the blazing Spanish sun.

A stocky, polite African American airman kept returning to sick call complaining of headaches, backaches and severe dizziness, after having been treated briefly with penicillin for gonorrhea. He was portrayed as a malingerer by the base surgeon as well as by his sergeant. One morning, he appeared on my list complaining of areas of visual loss. Using my newly obtained flight surgeon skills in perimetry and ocular examination, I discovered that he had severe retinitis. The back of the eye looked like a snowstorm. A lumbar puncture revealed a 4+ Mazzini test for syphilis in the spinal fluid. Although he had been treated for his initial gonorrhea, the brief course of penicillin had been insufficient to eradicate syphilis, which now infected his central nervous system.

We began treatment with high doses of intravenous penicillin, in a bed, in the base dispensary. That night, he shook terribly; his temperature increased to 106.4 with pulse rates of 150-175, and shock—a crisis due to the sudden death of the spirochetes circulating in his bloodstream. My experience with alcohol sponges was useful, but nonetheless, I sent him by ambulance to the El Cano Hospital where nurses were available to care for him. Colonel Morgan chuckled at my discomfort assuring me that this was classic "Jarisch-Herxheimer reaction." It would subside uneventfully and did just that. This was a lesson that all patient complaints, under any and all circumstances, must not be assumed to be psychological until all avenues of investigation have been exhausted.

An intolerant attitude was not confined to enlisted men. The base provost or sheriff, Major Woodruff, or Woody, a short potbellied man with a red neck and wattles, disliked me because I managed to finesse him at poker. One night, I folded my obvious flush to his hidden four-of-a-kind in a table stakes seven-card stud game. He actually tore up his cards and stormed out in a fury. Although accompanied by his wife in Spain, Woody made periodic sorties to the Ventas. He then appeared at the dispensary, sweating profusely, for penicillin injections, which I always dispensed without benefit of elaborate chart notes. So, our relationship remained friendly.

While living in the Bachelor Officers' Quarters, a civilian couple, the Richardses, regularly entertained me in their home. They were a delightful pair, a tall handsome civilian who headed personnel services and an ebullient French lady who also was a superb cook. Many evenings passed quickly. Richards taught me poker with serious diligence; we also matched wits at chess. I loved both of these attractive people for their kindness and their hospitality. One day, the provost and a small, quiet, ominous-looking CIA man arrived unannounced in my office at the base. They wanted to know everything about the Richardses and, in particular, details of any medical treatment that I had rendered. Woody, with this request, put his foot on my desk glaring threateningly while the dark spook slouched in a corner chair. I asked the CIA agent why they wanted to know these things. He said there had been a complaint by a local Spaniard. One or the other had fraternized "with a native" and both were to be declared *"persona non grata."* I had, in fact, treated them both medically, but for the most innocent and routine things. As I thought this over, I realized that, in addition to obvious intimidation, their request comprised a serious breach of ethics. The conversation had become patently outrageous.

"Woody, get your goddamned foot off of my desk!" He looked shocked and complied slowly. "These are fine people . . . I won't give you any medical information about any of my patients unless you take me to court." Woody jumped up, exclaiming furiously, his face even redder than ever, "Doc, I'll get you for this!" The CIA man frowned but said nothing. Then they both left. This unpleasant interchange occurred just before my wife arrived, and I, disturbed and frightened by that interview, warned her about answering questions about my friendship with this couple. I was sure I had done the right thing. Breaches of personal privacy then seemed common in government agencies. Now, with growing information databases, lapses in medical confidentiality are probably commonplace. A doctor cannot easily serve two masters, and, as pointed out by Major Woodruff, the government was paying me.

The same case can now be made for health maintenance organizations. It might be practical for patients, in some circumstances, to pay their physicians personally. For decades, the government has become quite concerned with protecting patient confidentiality, but such protection may be cosmetic.

After finishing the aviation medical course, I had second thoughts about surgery. I had hoped that, with the inauguration of the space program, I could compete for a position as an astronaut. After a year, it was clear that the bureaucratic vicissitudes of the space program, a stop-and-go enterprise, were such that this was an ephemeral goal. A brief flirtation occurred with Air France. I was invited to Paris to advise them on my capacity as a trained flight surgeon. They offered an executive position and a nice apartment in Paris. Friends of the Richardses who were executives in the airline had arranged this. They mainly wanted to know whether or not seats on Air France should be placed facing backward on the new jet aircraft and whether or not oxygen should be always used for high altitude flight. The French thought this might be a safer arrangement as on U.S. Air Force transports. I advised against it; passengers hated this arrangement, which was uncomfortable and, in any event, useless. If the plane crashed, there, inevitably, would be a high mortality. Placing seats backwards tended to emphasize this eventuality as remote as it might be. No commercial airline except the military transports had placed passenger seats facing backwards. The air force later abandoned this policy. Paris remained tempting, but the duties appeared insubstantial, almost trivial, compared to the challenges of surgical practice.

Along with my surgical duties, I now continued to fly in the F100-F to meet my hourly flight requirements. Later, the base got a squadron of F104s. Unfortunately, these Mach 2 fighters tended to crash. Four of my acquaintances were killed when these aircraft crashed. Nonetheless, I started to fly in the F104. It was a thrill to climb rapidly to 65,000 feet to the curvature of the earth and to a violet sky. These airplanes were enormously responsive, but with seven-foot wings, they fell like rocks with power loss. Lockheed technicians were permanently assigned to tinker and cure their various malfunctions. Later, after the German Air Force bought the F104s, these sophisticated craft continued their lethal history. I found being away from surgery to attend my flight duties taxing. I missed the operating room. I arranged to go to Madrid to scrub with the great consultant, Dr. Alton Ochsner, who periodically visited the main base hospital. I would work up his patients; and then start operating very early in the morning. The local surgeons did not enjoy working with him since he was considered demanding. I later learned that he trained Dr. Michael DeBakey. As a third year medical student, Dr. De Bakey, while being questioned by Ochsner, was rumored to have once fainted in the amphitheater (the bullpen) at Tulane. As a tough Bronx kid, I remained oblivious to his innuendoes and pointed questions. He insisted that everything be tied with cotton. He made large incisions. He operated slowly, but recognizing my good fortune, I worked with him at every opportunity. He was an absolute master at exposing pathology and correcting problems in a logical and safe way. The most difficult cases were saved for him to operate upon.

At 7:00 A.M. one day, he made a large transverse incision in the upper abdomen of an obese warrant officer. We were operating for a deeply placed peptic ulcer eroding into the common duct leading from the liver. He then extended the excision up to the epigastrium and lower chest in the shape of a "T." By most standards, this case was exceedingly difficult; this was exactly the reason why the regular air force surgeon had it saved for Dr. Ochsner. By 1:00 P.M., he had finished a common bile duct repair and a gastric resection. He asked me close the T-shaped incision with interrupted cotton sutures. I was having a hard enough time just tying the cotton he insisted upon using for hemostasis. As soon as Ochsner left the room, the sergeant scrub technician winked. He handed me a long piece of nylon on a big needle. I closed expeditiously with a continuous suture, then went to the locker room for a shower. Sprawled out naked on the bench in the steamy room, I was smoking a cigarette when the master surgeon walked into the haze. His eyes widened in surprise, almost in disbelief. With a look of angry contempt, he silently turned and strode out without a word. I figured he knew I could not have closed the wound that rapidly with interrupted cotton. He announced a grand rounds conference with all the hospital staff that afternoon. He told all assembled that if anybody smoked again in front of him, he would leave the base. I was relieved that he said nothing about my choice of wound closure. To my relief, the large incision healed uneventfully. Dr. Ochsner was far ahead of his time in recognizing the connection between cigarette smoking and lung cancer. All of us at that time smoked cigarettes and, regrettably, continued to do so for many more years, before we acknowledged the obvious connection.

As the base population grew to more than 6,000 souls, it turned out that, in addition to my regular night duty, I was out about every third night taking care of one or another surgical emergency. Fracture work was common. Fortunately, I was well trained in this specialty as a medical student at Bellevue Hospital and as a junior resident at Presbyterian Hospital. Here, too, the store of books in the footlocker proved invaluable. I did appendectomies, operations on gall bladders, and repaired several perforated ulcers. Six months after my tour began, my wife, Eve, arrived. We set up housekeeping on Calle Ascuncion in the Triana. It was a beautiful time. For the first time, we had enough money, and help, in the way of a delightful but eccentric household servant, Dolores Avril. I had employed her through Antonio the Portero, the janitor of the building, when I went to rent the apartment. He offered me, with a leer, a young and handsome woman (*muy joven* and *guapa*). I said, "Absolutely not." I wanted one that was *vieja y gorda*. Dolores, old and fat, took great care of us. However, she was basically a *niñera*, a helper with children. We will always love her. But dinner parties with her serving the table were unpredictable events. She could never manage the requisite white gloves. She carried on a kind of running conversation with Spanish guests, breaking any kind of formal mood, which was supposed to prevail for these occasions. She insisted on telling them what good people we were. One night, I heard some unusually loud high-pitched feminine argument from the kitchen. My wife had discovered that the whipped cream for the "Great American Strawberry Shortcake," a treat for Spanish dignitaries, had become salad dressing.

My interests in aviation as a flight surgeon and in general surgery as the base surgeon divided my time. I found that I could not afford to take much leave. Colonel Morgan, in his diffident way, asked me to stay available on a twenty-four-hour basis. I did not accept his request with the grace that I should have. But it was true that, every time I was absent, there was an adverse incident or later missed event.

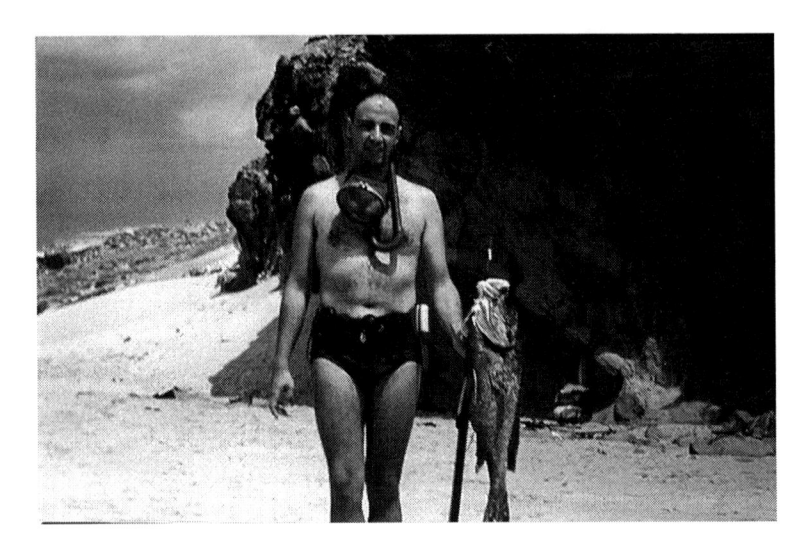

Fishing at Tarifa, Spain

I was able to take short fishing trips. Upon returning from a short weekend respite, I would find some unusual cast applications by our contract surgeons. These always required some type of revision. The local populace showed the effects of unskilled orthopedic care: many limping people with deformed limbs, probably due to misplaced fractures. In order to progress in orthopedics, I took lessons from Jose Maria Cortez, a master orthopedic surgeon. He relied almost solely on closed reduction of fractures, fearing introduction of osteomyelitis with open techniques. I learned the trick of closed reductions of both bones of the forearm with a compression splint. Usually, these required open operation. When I saw a muscular man with such a fracture, I informed Jose that we might reduce this easily. He taught me a lesson that I never learned as well as I should have: "Rafael, do you know how to catch flies?" As I stared blankly, he said, "Open your mouth." Fortunately, our closed reductions were quite successful. The Spaniards were full of wise aphorisms, for example, "The scalded cat flees from cold water." Ultimately, by the time of my discharge, I had accumulated sixty days of leave with no vacation, a pattern, like that of the scalded cat, that I continued for years.

As my aviation education continued, I took flying lessons and soloed the aero club's Cessna 150 after six hours of instruction by Colonel Godman, the base commander. I had some dangerous experiences as a novice flyer. On one occasion, I was sent to Gibraltar in the Cessna 150 for the local liquor run for the officers' club. The airplane was loaded while I went to town to look into some English tailoring and a long lunch. I returned at 1:00 P.M. on a hot afternoon. Boxes of liquor were tidily stowed aft of the cockpit seats. I figured, thoughtlessly, that everyone knew what was to be done in properly loading the airplane. But whether sailing, flying or in surgery, assumptions are always dangerous. After clearance, I pushed the throttle all the way in. The tiny craft rolled and rolled down the runway but did not take off at the usual distance. The plane had obviously been overloaded. I just got off the end of the runway. Flying dead into an east wind over the choppy strait of Gibraltar, I slowly gained enough altitude to climb over the Sierra to my home base.

My flight instructor, a highly disciplined Strategic Air Command officer was a tough but fair man. He had been the personal pilot of General McArthur and was a close personal friend of General LeMay. A perfectionist, he was highly critical when I passed my written pilot's examination with an 85% grade. "I hope you're better at medicine, Doc." The little Cessna felt quite like a freed bird when this large man got out to tell me to solo for the first time. One day, I noticed, after the Cessna had been serviced, unequal magneto drops on the engine run up. One side was slightly below minimums. I called the tower to let them know. The colonel happened to be there and radioed, "Well, Doc, it's all right." I accelerated down the wide, long SAC runway and, at 400 feet of altitude, the engine just quit and froze. Rather than landing into the wind and the olive grove directly ahead, I executed a 180-degree turn. The light craft floated back downwind over the runway with three bounces on touchdown. It was not pretty, but it was a landing. Any landing you walk away from is supposed to be a good landing. The choice was to clip the grove or the downwind landing. It was, in fact, exactly the wrong thing. Colonel Godman was furious. He insisted that I learn dead stick landings in small spaces. I had to practice for hours on a small tract that he had specially cleared out in another olive grove. After all, who wants an 85% doctor or pilot? I later learned that the piston rings had been installed upside down, which had caused the engine freeze-up. But nothing was said about this. I still have nightmares about doing landings and takeoffs in small spaces.

Pressure grew for me to stay in the air force as a flight surgeon. I enjoyed the company of the fliers and their esprit de corps. An opportunity arose to serve on temporary duty to Nellis Air Force Base near Las Vegas to learn about the health hazards of tritium leaks from hydrogen bombs. I needed a top-secret clearance and to get it, I reported to a security agency in a shack on the base. Here, the civilian spook type, Woody's CIA friend, gleefully had me complete a massive array of forms. At the age of twenty-seven, I was required to name all my girlfriends for the past ten years. That was a tough assignment. I did not know why, but the prevailing opinion in the FBI at the time of Hoover was that we were not supposed to be screwing girls. Of course, we now all know what the director himself was doing. Between the ages of sixteen and twenty-five, New York kids were active. I had been married a little over two years and worried about complying with this request. I knew that I would risk life and limb in betraying the confidences of former girlfriends, particularly New York Irish or Italian ladies. Both the base and the hospital commanders called, "Please, just give them a few names." That done, I quickly put the matter out of my mind.

During the time when we were back in the United States, several young women called my mother's home in Yonkers. They told her of men in dark suits, white shirts, and sunglasses appearing at their doorsteps with pointed inquiries. Luckily, they appartently harbored no hard feelings. I asked Toni O'Neal what she said, and she replied, "I told them you are a good guy as did several others." The top-secret clearance was granted. I went to Nellis Air Base in Nevada. During this terrifying interlude, I learned what happens when radioactive tritium gets into total body water. As a matter of fact, those several weeks in Las Vegas and the tritiated water horror convinced me that I wanted nothing to do with nuclear energy. Benjamin Spock and Linus Pauling soon courageously spoke out against nuclear power, but it took three decades for most responsible leaders to concur. The paranoia of the Cold War, so terrifying then, seemed distant until the recent crises between India and Pakistan. I remember that some of the people I encountered in the atomic establishment were as scary and weird as *Dr. Strangelove.*

Sampling life in Las Vegas and living in that colorful city was an interesting experience. What made it most interesting was how lively and friendly the place was, all the while we knew that nearby resided the wherewithal to destroy the planet. I felt, then, that I would come back to that vivid lively town. I was relieved to return to Seville, and friends took us out to celebrate my return and another reunion with Eve. Some friends gave us a flamenco party at The Venta De Bajo. We drank Jerez, strong sherry, and clapped to the counterpoint. I came to love the flamenco rhythms of the Sevillanas during *feria* and the haunting melodic *saetas* of Holy Week. The party was a mistake. I got a call from Colonel Morgan at 4:00 A.M. just after falling into an almost comatose sleep. There had been an airplane crash. I told the colonel that I had been drinking. "Well," he said in his quiet drawl, "we know that because the air police spotted you. We will send the ambulance out to get you. Don't drive out to the hospital. The cook is here. You will have breakfast and coffee and scrambled eggs." After that fine breakfast, I was able to reduce two open fractures and remove a spleen. The meal and youthful hepatic metabolism saved the day. This was absolutely the last time I ever drank when likely to be called for surgical emergencies. Later in my career as chief of surgery, I dealt with this problem when complaints arose about surgical staff members apparently under the influence. There could be no compromise and suspensions with counseling were mandatory. Later, drug usage had to be added into this unpleasant equation.

My career indecision continued, with the prospect of a regular commission in the air force and a career in aviation medicine. Then, several things conspired to change my mind. One was the departure of Colonel Morgan, who was replaced by a fat, pompous major from New Mexico. With a silly grin, he told me that my next assignment as a regular officer would probably be a missile silo somewhere in Nebraska. This obnoxious man knew nothing about medicine and provoked near rebellion by insisting that all officers have Christmas dinner in the hospital. My love affair with the air force related to the aviators and a kind West Texan doctor. This type of "support personnel" some called "base weenies." I now became aware of this distinction as I contemplated an air force career. The prospects of continued association with base weenies, and even becoming one myself were unpalatable. The main thing that changed my mind was that, while we sojourned in the United States, my wife had gotten pregnant.

Our first son was born in Seville amidst great celebration. Friends and neighbors gathered outside of our terrace to sing, "*Rafaelito de mi corazon*, Ralph of my heart." Dolores Avril was in her glory as a *niñera*. She certainly helped launch our son to the right way. As a new father, continued F104 crashes gave me an inkling of my own mortality and responsibilities. I needed to get a residency position and searched the country for training, particularly in vascular surgery. Unfortunately, topnotch training was not available in a military residency at this time.

A beautiful young woman, a warrant officer's wife, brought this lesson home. She had appeared to ask my nurse for blood pressure medication. She reported that she had been seen by many doctors at many base facilities and just wanted a medication refill. She did not want an examination, and did not want to wait for me to see her. I insisted on interviewing her and was glad that I did so. She suffered from intractable headaches due to high blood pressure and had been told that there was nothing to be done. She was facing her early death with quiet resignation. She reiterated that all she wanted was a refill of her blood pressure medication, and reluctantly submitted to physical examination. Her blood pressure was 220/120, but her groin pulses were barely palpable. Over the thoracic aorta, there was a harsh murmur characteristic of coarctation, a congenital narrowing of this main artery. I told her she needed an operation. While searching for a referral site, she ultimately had to be sent to the Mayo Clinic—not an air force hospital. That settled the issue for me. I would seek the best training in vascular surgery available. After her operation, I watched her dancing at the Officers Club with her husband; they kissed just as the music stopped, a satisfying outcome of a routine physical examination. As the last weeks wound down, I treated several severe trauma cases, including penetrating abdominal wounds. I left Spain with sadness but also with relief. In spite of my inexperience, there had been no major complications or deaths; it is probably better to be lucky than good. And I had been lucky.

So I returned to New York, something I did not really want to do. I was now thirty years of age with a new son. I resumed junior residency duties, working every other night for $50 a month while wearing a silly white high-necked uniform. On the positive side, I got laundry service and all the food I could eat. The chief of surgery made room for me in the over-crowded residency. Dr. Harold Zintel took mercy on me when I made an urgent flight on New Year's Eve back to the United States to ask for the residency appointment I had previously neglected to accept. The lowest point in my new life occurred when one of my fellow interns, who had skipped the service and finished his training in ophthalmology, appeared one evening in a velvet-collared Brooks Brothers overcoat. He now had a Park Avenue practice. I was scurrying around on the wards drawing bloods and starting intravenous infusions dressed in the silly Dr. Kildare shirt. He was pleasant but aloof. He snickered as he told me he had avoided "signing up for anything" and had not been drafted. He had pioneered in techniques for dealing with diabetic retinopathy, a major contribution. I, on the other hand, had simply frittered away three years. It became obvious to me that the road to success involved innovation and advancing the art and science of medicine. Reliance upon governmental beneficence always involved attached strings.

In response to a series of incomprehensible letters from Air Force Reserve, Denver, Colorado, I resigned my commission as soon as I had served six years. This instinctive decision was fortunate. Had I not resigned, I never would have had a career in academic surgery. President Kennedy called reserve officers up for the Berlin crisis, and this is exactly why an academic position at Western Reserve became available.

The three years in Spain were a surgical audition, and combined with that New York year, I felt I had been through an inquisition that strengthened commitment to surgery. My capabilities had been tested, but I had fallen far behind the rest of my colleagues. This became apparent when I worked for my former interns as a junior resident. I did not accomplish this as gracefully as I should have, though they clearly knew more than I did. After reading most of the major surgical journals spanning the three years of my absence, it became clear that I had developed an inflated idea of my knowledge base. I had treated a population of young and healthy people and had not been confronted with the sick elderly. The result of any slight misstep with old, sick patients was lethal and my ideas about fluid management were outmoded. In spite of my own shortcomings, I was dissatisfied with the overall quality of surgery and surgical education then practiced in New York City. This negative attitude infected my thinking and work, in spite of the fact that St. Luke's was the first to succeed at open heart and major vascular surgery in New York. The three years in Spain had convinced me that I could be an effective surgeon. But I really was not as good as I had thought I was. The audition had gone well in my mind, but my future was uncertain. I thought it perhaps presumptuous to believe that I could ever be a surgeon.

JOURNEY TO THE WESTERN RESERVE

> But when you journey, leave behind
> The bigot's stern unsocial mind.
>
> Moses Warren: The Explorer's Farewell

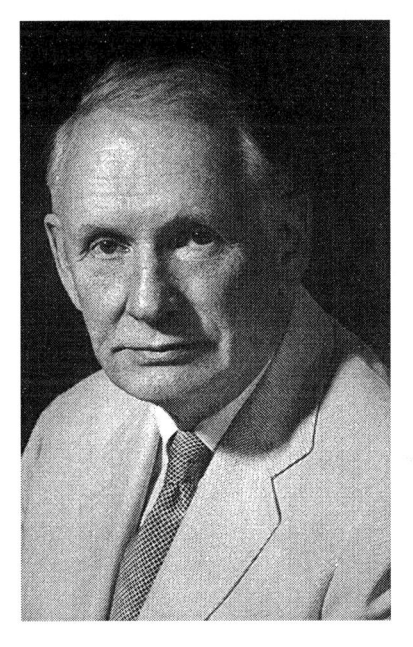

William D Holden, MD, FACS

After military service, my choices were limited. Remaining in New York City involved at least a year in research before completing surgical training at St. Luke's, or I could move to another, probably inferior, residency. Having left St. Luke's program for military service, I was not in line with their five-year rotation, and I had not had the foresight to plan a return. I was not sure if I wanted to continue after my second year, so I went to Spain and made no plans to return. My own lack of foresight and ambivalence about surgical residency led to the lowest point in my life up to this time. Now that I was eager to complete surgical training, particularly after three years of lagging behind my intern class, I had no job. I was impatient to get on with clinical work, rather than marking time in a dog lab. Having flirted with beguiling alternative careers, I now paid the price for a lack of constancy. December 1961 in New York was cold and dark; rain alternated with a nasty sleet. I received the dismal news that I could not go directly into a rotation next year, and would have to spend a year, possibly two years, in research. Living in Yonkers and commuting by car to Manhattan was exasperating. Bruckner Boulevard, that miserable stretch of road through the Bronx, always under construction, came to symbolize all the ugliness and inconvenience of New York City.

A resident, a year senior to me at that time, offered pivotal advice. Dr. William Reid, an outspoken critic of deficiencies in the New York surgical scene and surgical education, advised me to leave the training program. Opinions about Bill could be harsh because of his outspoken cynicism, but he had a keen unerring diagnostic sense. It is important to listen to these blunt people, even though, because of a brutal honesty, they may appear eccentric. Such individuals can be unpopular and politically incorrect. But for me, at that time, Bill's counsel was direct and on the mark. When an opportunity arose for a residency position at my level at Western Reserve in Cleveland, he urged me to go there. He himself had been interviewed by the chief of surgery, Dr. Holden. Surprisingly, he characterized Holden as a "saint." Saint, indeed. I had not thought Dr. Reid to be capable of even harboring such a sentiment. Dr. Reid's assessment was highly accurate; William D. Holden ultimately exerted a profound influence on my life, as he did upon the lives of many others. Because of his charisma, Holden was later characterized as a "sage," a "prophet," and as the embodiment of the Greek spirit "agape."

After completing my morning rounds at 5:00 A.M., I retrieved my car in the parking lot and drove in the dark from Manhattan to Newark Airport. The little Volkswagen skidded erratically on the bridges of the icy New Jersey Turnpike. I had an appointment in Cleveland early that afternoon. The flight was uneventful, and I took a cab to the east side of Cleveland, arriving there before noon. After lunch in the Cleveland Museum of Art, I had time to view some spectacular exhibits, and then, I jogged, through bitter cold, to University Hospitals, a massive array of buildings on Adelbert Road and Euclid Avenue. The hospital entrance replicated that of the Peter Bent Brigham Hospital; I wondered whether this imitation was accidental or deliberate. An old-fashioned elevator hand operated by a pleasant black lady lifted us to the seventh floor. Curiously, there were two hand-operated doors, one opening into the operating room hall, the other leading directly into an antique oak-paneled outer office, which was the Department of Surgery. I learned that the door to the office had been the private entrance of a former chief, Dr. Elliott Cutler, who became the chief at the Peter Bent Brigham Hospital in Boston. Apparently, Dr. Cutler liked entering and leaving unobserved. This door was no longer used.

Within the office, an attractive blond lady, Miss Jean Klippert, presided over yet another paneled inner sanctum. After a pleasant welcome, she led me into, dark, oak-paneled office. Dr. Holden was sitting at a desk with a lamp illuminating his work area and his head and shoulders. He was a spare, ascetic-appearing, gray-haired man with sharp piercing blue eyes, which were at once curious and sensitive. His demeanor appeared exceedingly controlled, even to the point of mildness, yet, he projected unquestioned authority. This unusual man was unlike any surgeon that I had encountered before. He asked pointed questions about past experience and my goals and ambitions. He seemed bemused by the fact that I was from the Bronx. Abruptly, he queried, "When can you come?" "Well, sir, I have obligations in New York." His reply was almost a low growl, "I'll take care of that." We settled on July 1. The return flight and the slipping-and-sliding drive to Yonkers left me wondering why I had so quickly agreed. Even for me, this was a very sudden decision; I felt practically seduced. Over supper that night back in Yonkers, I told my mother and stunned wife with babe in her arms that we were to move to Cleveland in July.

For six months in New York, I remained in my lame duck residency in funny high-collared "Dr. Kildare" uniforms. I had hated these from the start, feeling somehow stigmatized. According to the resident handbook, our white shoes were to be kept "suitably polished." This discipline was reasonable, but the pompous instructions had always offended me. Why would someone have dirty shoes while tending to patients? I wanted to leave New York immediately. The chief at St. Luke's, who had been my advocate all along, dissuaded me from taking this impetuous step. I later discovered that this good man was having his own problems with his position. He left shortly to become an official of the American College of Surgeons.

Six months passed quickly. Much of my operating time was assigned with Richard B. Stark in plastic surgery. The senior residents preferred abdominal cases that were considered more major. That attitude always puzzled me; surgery was surgery, whether of the eyes, or the bones or the skin. Many of the cases that were done on Stark's service were quite major, including cleft lips and palates and radical facial reconstructions for bone injuries. From this kind master surgeon and artist, I learned precise tissue handling and gentleness. He gradually had me do more and more complex parts of his procedures. That spring, Dr. Stark suggested that I begin training in plastic surgery with him, but vascular disease and sick patients continued to fascinate me, and I felt that I had to prove myself in general surgery before specializing. As mild as Stark was, like all great surgeons, he was an unrelenting taskmaster. One evening, rushing through the hospital lobby to my wife who was idling our car in a no-parking zone, I felt Stark eyeing me with concern. I turned to ask, "What is the problem, Dr. Stark?" We had just completed a large flap procedure on an ulcerated leg that required an extensive immobilizing splint. The splint was effective, but I had rushed the application. It was bulky and unattractive. "Well," he said gently, "the splint you put on is not your usual work." I returned to reapply a neat splint and slept that night in our call room.

Plastic surgery became a welcome refuge from the chaos of general surgery. The procedures were done on schedule and carefully preplanned, something that seemed not to occur in general abdominal surgery. I seriously considered a career change, but it was hard to tell whether this was because of the quiet competence of Stark himself and my fondness for him or because of the work. An interchange involving Stark and one of his rhinoplasty patients finally made up my mind about a career in plastic surgery. One Sunday morning on rounds, we removed a nose splint from a New York rhinoplasty patient. Carefully peeling away the tape and fine plaster, we unveiled the usual upturned pert nose along with the customary black-and-blue raccoon eyes. The nose looked very good to me. Upon peering into her mirror, the young woman burst into tears. She berated our work, doctors in general, herself for being such a fool and finally, the ever patient Stark. "I am undone," were her final words. In spite of our efforts to console her, she wept hysterically. Finally, Stark uttered in a low pleading voice, "Please, Miss Weiner, it is Sunday." I could never have been so patient. Cosmetic surgery was not for me. Stark persisted in trying to convert me; if I did not like cosmetic surgery, there was always "reconstructive" plastic surgery.

On June 29, I was still working with no respite from the call schedule. June 30, 1962 was the day I allotted for driving to my new position in Cleveland. I crossed the George Washington Bridge on a hot and muggy afternoon, and then drove south to the New Jersey Highway, and then, west on Pennsylvania Turnpike. The fresh breeze here was pleasant. I needed to report on July 1 in Cleveland, so there were no rest stops. That afternoon, my Volkswagen's radio could only pick up country-western music. There was no WQXR. Perhaps, I thought, I should never have gone west of the Hudson. A left turn off Route 80 led me, at midnight, into the Flats of Cleveland. Here was a vision of hell: smoke, smell, and blazing steel furnaces. Greeted by all of the things that made this city so wealthy, yet, which made it, on first sight, unattractive, I began to worry. Then I drove along an oily river, the Cuyahoga, that river later famous for catching on fire. I turned east on Euclid Avenue, which took me to the house officers' quarters called Robb House at two in the morning. As I learned later, there were better and more scenic ways to enter the City of Cleveland. I was to live in that dormitory for four months while I waited for the family to move.

The first day was not propitious, either. I, apparently, was not expected that night and there was no room for me there. I needed ten dollars for a bed at the University Inn. Perhaps, I thought, Dr. Holden had forgotten he had hired me. More likely, someone else had forgotten. At the crack of dawn, I headed straight for Lakeside, to the seventh floor. Drs. Holden and Charles Hubay, his gentle Hungarian associate, looked worried. I had been assigned first to pediatric surgery and, as it was put diplomatically, to "a demanding surgeon and demanding service." I was relieved to have a job. "Don't worry, I'll manage," crossed my mind as I thought of my previous experiences with Dr. Alton Ochsner. I was promptly introduced to Dr. Robert Izant, the "Big I" as he was called by generations of residents. Trained by Dr. Gross of Boston and descended from an old Cleveland family, he regarded me suspiciously through demilunar glasses perched low on his nose. I guessed he had never worked with anyone from the Bronx before.

I went to work and did not leave Robb House or the hospital for six weeks. The pediatric surgery service flourished with the help of an elegant St. Luke's nurse—all starch, discipline and confidence. She had somehow migrated to Cleveland and still wore her distinctive cap. Dr. Izant was to become a lifelong friend and supporter. He later operated on my youngest daughter. Pediatric surgery was a challenge, but the gentle techniques absorbed from Stark were of great help when it came to repairing congenital lesions in tiny infants. Dr. Izant and his associate, Dr.Robert Miller, were totally dedicated to the care of sick babies. All of us were in awe of Dr. Izant's abilities. We feared his tongue and tolerated his occasional tantrums, which really were more show than substance.

Dr. Holden could not tolerate slow or dilatory operating. On occasion, he would actually start cases for chronic offenders who were late going to the operating room. His office was immediately down the hall from the operating suites. He seemed to know if all rooms were not off and running at 8:00 A.M. sharp. In the pediatric surgery room, which was preferentially warmed to 80 degrees, his head appeared at the door at 8:10. An eight-month-old infant with bilateral hernias lay on the table, anesthetized, awaiting the arrival of the "Big I." We were scrubbed, gowned, and ready. The baby was well wrapped to prevent heat loss. Holden's deep-voiced inquiry brought us all to attention. "What are you doing?" "Hernias, sir, waiting for Dr. Izant." The voice, in an even lower tone commanded, "Please get started." I had expected that another attending would come to assist, but no one appeared. Fortunately, I had done many pediatric hernias during my rotation in Spain. By 8:25 A.M., I was on the second side when Dr. Izant sauntered in, joking, as was usual, with the nursing team. I sensed his initial angry response when he saw what was going on. Then came a chuckle, "You might as well finish." And he left the room. The circulating nurse had whispered word of the professor's visit. No secrets exist in operating suites. Later, when I became a young attending, Dr. Izant gave me the privilege of covering pediatric surgery when he was out of town.

The surgical environment in Cleveland was, in many ways, in order of magnitude, better than that of New York. Dr. Holden had gathered a unique faculty. In addition to Dr. Charles Hubay, there were Dr. John Davis, vascular surgeon thought to be the model for "Hawkeye" in the "Mash" television series, Dr. William Abbott, a gastric surgeon and distinguished researcher, Dr. William Drucker, who was defining the biochemistry and physiology of shock, and Dr. Jack Cole, who was studying the peculiar transformation of colon polyps into cancer. Dr. Jay Ankeney was already miles ahead in cardiac surgery. The resident, a year ahead of me, Dr. Donald Gann, was an established investigator, and with Dr. Hastings K. Wright, was elaborating the neuroendocrine sequelae of shock in the laboratories.

The monk, Rabelais, a surgeon himself, had written of an ideal place, the Abbe of Theleme. There, no one unpleasant, boring or ugly was allowed. At that time, at least it seemed to me, these were magical people in a magical place, another Theleme, in the Western Reserve of Ohio. I was happy there. In sharp contrast to relationships with New Yorkers, my dealings with Ohioans constantly amazed me. Midwesterners, in general, appeared quite relaxed and, yet, they projected energy at the same time. They spoke with calm flat voices with never a histrionic emphasis to be heard. That faculty's impact on the resident staff was electric and never forgotten by any of us. All respected basic science ability, but clinical excellence was a first priority; whereas, in the East, some trainees were clearly destined to be rat and mouse doctors. This attitude, exactly, had conditioned my initial lack of desire to spend time in the laboratory during clinical training. Fortunately, I was to have that opportunity later. Cleveland surgeons were, for the most part, distinctly better technicians than many of the surgeons I had encountered in New York. They were competent, rapid operators, always pleasant and apparently relaxed.

In contrast to the New York situation, money appeared to be of little concern to them. For the average Park Avenue surgeon, at least at that time, an ideal patient would be an anorexic ninety-five pound heiress with obvious uncomplicated appendicitis. I am being unfair in this pronouncement, as I had worked with some outstanding New York surgeons, particularly at St. Luke's. But on the average, messy or troublesome cases seen in the emergency room where I interned were likely to be "LCH'd," or sent to the local city hospital. A patient's lack of funds guaranteed the transfer to a city hospital, though exceptions existed, particularly with the younger surgeons on staff at St. Luke's.

Early in my Cleveland experience, I saw a terribly complicated vascular case for Dr. John Davis late on a Friday night. He had had three prior procedures and this was his third graft failure. He was an indigent patient who could not afford to pay fees for the extensive surgery required to save his leg. I asked if I should inquire about sending the patient across town to the County Hospital, where

Dr. Simeone had a vascular service. John Davis' eyes widened in surprise, "What on earth for? This is a 'tasty' case." That attitude was pervasive among our staff. Difficult cases were not problems but challenges to be met happily, and we were successful in saving this man's leg. Had I admitted such a messy indigent case in New York, I would have been in deep trouble.

Four chief residents staffed the university hospital and the Veterans Hospital on the west side in Brecksville. We were required to stay in-house every other night and were always on call for our own services, and through it all, we remained colleagues, not competitors. A laid-back Midwest charitable attitude made room for Bronx brashness, as well as for an Italian proclivity to be loud and too outspoken. If these Midwesterners were critical of my ways, they were thoughtful as well as kind, though one of the senior faculty said, "You can take the boy out of the city, but you can't take the city out of the boy." I did try hard to change, to tone myself down, but I remained unsparingly critical of my own shortcomings and publicly critical of any inadequacy in patient care.

I write this account three decades later in a bright academic office in Reno, Nevada, while I scrutinize two of Robert Izant's remarkable watercolors on the opposite wall. One is a luminous view of Mason Street from Vallejo in San Francisco, and the other, an all-brown and dirty view of the Cuyahoga River, the river in Cleveland Flats that actually burned. Dr. Holden died in 1996, aged eighty-one years. His obituary, written by Dr. Jack Cole said, "Those of us whose good fortune it was to work under and with Bill will remember him as a dignified and gentle man who neither browbeat nor belittled in his efforts to bring out the best in us. He was survived by his three children, two brothers, a sister, seven grandchildren and his dear friend, Jean Klippert."

My journey west of the Hudson to the Western Reserve during the Holden era, Halcyon years, was a stroke of extreme good fortune for me. In the year that I was to finish residency, Miss Klippert summoned me to the oak-paneled office. In the spring of 1964, Dr. Abbott had died suddenly of severe coronary disease. Dr.

Holden, sitting at his desk, was writing under that same lamp illuminating his work in that dark office. He looked up, thoughtfully saying, "I hear you might like this academic stuff." "Yes! Yes, sir." The voice, an octave lower again, said, "Do you want to stay?" My heart leapt. "Yessir!" He shuffled some papers, then said, "Well, you will get ten thousand dollars a year and, of course, secretarial help. All right?" "Yessir!"

I had joined an abbey in mid-America. What young man from the wilds of the Bronx could have had such fortune? My doubts about surgery and my own abilities to do it well were all resolved in that place. Now, many years later, faced with a difficult decision as a chief myself, I close my eyes tightly—a gesture of Holden's when he was deep in thought. I try not to be impulsive and to think about what he would have done, or did, when faced with a similar problem.

AN EASY LIFE: CLEVELAND CASES

> The humility which comes from others having faith in you.
> Dag Hammarskjold

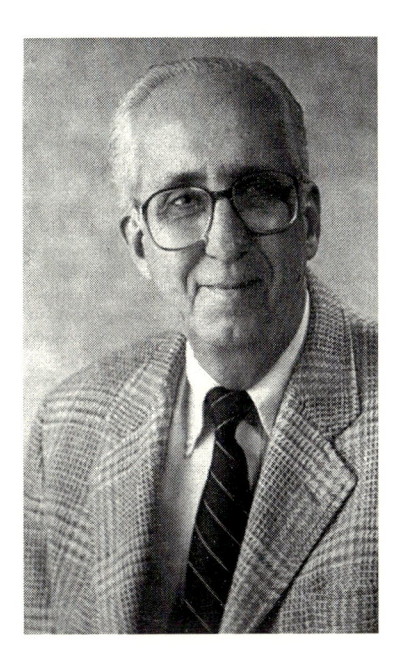

Charles A Hubay, MD, FACS

A chief residency in surgery once granted young surgeons virtually total responsibility for patient care, and this experience changed our lives. University Hospitals of Cleveland in the 1960s had two services of 35 beds solely for staff patients, each ward supervised by a chief surgical resident. Each service had priorities for elective surgery on alternate days and we examined patients in our own clinics every second day. Residents were entirely responsible for guiding patients' work-ups, admissions, treatment, and follow-up. Each chief had two assistant residents, an intern, and several medical students. Attending surgeons scrubbed on staff cases only when invited, and usually to demonstrate some special expertise. That year was exhilarating. We grew in knowledge and experience, and our technical abilities increased exponentially under a heavy caseload of operative procedures. From one week to the next, each of us grew into a more expert clinician and, in other ways, into a more disciplined person.

Cleveland had always been an important center for thyroid surgery. A paucity of iodine in the Midwestern diet had caused thyroid disease. The senior Dr. George Crile, a former chairman at University Hospitals, had pioneered thyroid surgery, and the institution had accumulated extensive experience in treating thyroid disorders. Another former chief of surgery at Western Reserve, Dr. Lenhart, along with Dr. Marine, then introduced iodized salt as prophylaxis. While the prevalence of goiter decreased throughout the Midwest, thyroid disease was still a relatively common surgical problem. We had, as junior residents, developed considerable experience assisting at and performing thyroidectomy. We did not regard thyroid procedures to be as challenging as gastrectomy or aneurysm repair.

Although I should have known better, I learned that thyroid surgery is no routine matter; no surgery ever is. There is no such thing as a minor case. We had scheduled Ozzie Jones, a charming thirty-nine-year-old African American lady, for an operation to remove a solitary nodule in the left lobe of her thyroid gland. At that time, we depended upon palpation; ultrasound was not then available. The rapid appearance and growth of this nodule indicated surgical intervention. We operated on Mrs. Jones at the end of a long schedule after a gastrectomy and two biliary procedures. After exposing the left thyroid lobe, we found a soft cyst protruding from the front of the gland. The cyst was well localized and could be removed easily by partial thyroid lobectomy. The teaching at that time was than such cysts are benign and not cancerous. I placed a neat rosette of Crile clamps, excised the cyst with a rim of normal thyroid tissue and handed it to the pathologist who opened the specimen in the room. The cavity was filled with a whitish fluid. The pathologist pronounced the cyst benign, which was good news at the end of a long day. I asked for a frozen section and the verdict was, again, that the process was benign. The junior resident urged me to go ahead, and complete a thyroid lobectomy. He was always in favor of more, rather than less, surgery. Regardless of the timing, total lobectomy carried real additional risks to the patient, such as nerve or parathyroid damage. Partial excision was then accepted treatment for such a lesion. Two days later, we discharged a happy Mrs. Jones.

A week later, after there had been time for scarring to occur, the pathologist called to tell me he had found malignancy within the cyst. Our operation had been inadequate. I went to see Dr. Hubay, and he, in his characteristically gentle way, told me that I needed to reoperate, to remove the left lobe totally, as well as the opposite thyroid lobe. I whined, complaining, "That's not going to be easy." Dr. Hubay looked at me and replied, "I never told you it would be an easy life." I learned a great deal that day.

Mrs. Jones took the news of the need for another operation with remarkably good grace. The procedure, as expected, proved to be difficult because of dense scarring. But we had been taught to always identify the recurrent laryngeal nerves and parathyroid glands. Dr. Hubay looked in, from time to time, to observe our progress but did not offer to scrub. Damage to the nerves could result in hoarseness, while parathyroid deficiency could result in severe muscular spasms. The operation proceeded slowly and with deliberation. It turned out that the cancer had all been removed from the left lobe at the initial operation, but other small foci of cancer were discovered on the right. The patient recovered uneventfully, and Ozzie and her husband appeared grateful in spite of our need to reoperate. As the couple was leaving, they told us that they owned a bar, really a "sporting house," close to Lakeside Hospital on Carnegie Avenue.

They invited us to a party to celebrate her successful operation, and our resident team and medical students all attended. I was initially dubious about visiting a sporting house, whatever that meant, but that evening turned out to be a memorable occasion, with a Motown jazz band, ribs, drinks, and prayers. We were offered favors of the house, which, of course, we declined. I said to a beautiful young woman who came to sit next to me at the bar that this was one of the best parties I had ever seen, and I had seen many. She laughed and whispered into my ear, "There is nothing better than being black on a Saturday night in Cleveland." I had the privilege of treating Ozzie and her husband for miscellaneous illnesses during two decades in Cleveland. They were loyal patients and regularly sought my advice for other medical problems over the years. Mrs. Jones had no recurrence of her thyroid cancer, and the sporting house, to the best of my knowledge, continued to prosper until I left Cleveland. Ozzie and her husband then became patients of Dr. Hubay.

In 1964, exciting new surgical procedures were being developed. The decade of the '60s saw the birth of vascular surgery, and Cleveland played an important role in this development. Dr. Frank Spencer, then of Kentucky, had popularized partition of the vena cava, the large vein within the abdomen, as a means of preventing migration of clots from the legs into the lungs. The procedure required mobilizing the cava just below the renal veins, and then placing sutures front to back and side to side to create a sort of silk screen within the vein. The operation was indicated when pulmonary emboli occurred in spite of anticoagulation. My senior resident associate, Dr. Tim Corday, and I had seen several patients die with recurrent pulmonary emboli and we went to see Dr. Holden, the chief, for his views. We believed we should offer this operation since this was a lethal problem. No attending surgeon was enthusiastic about helping us perform this new procedure. Dr. Holden gave us permission to assist each other on properly selected cases. The first three cases went smoothly, but during the fourth case, we tore the back wall of the vena cava just as we passed a large clamp around the vessel to control it. Massive audible bleeding followed this event, and bleeding which can be heard is quickly lethal. We both recognized the immediate danger to the life of our patient. We could lose the patient on the operating table; this is not, or hardly ever, an acceptable event. Jim was a calm competent surgeon, but he had a cast in his right eye which wandered outward and appeared when he was excited or distressed. As I looked across the table, I saw that his lazy eye had wandered outward to a considerable degree, more than I had ever seen before.

Somehow, Dr. William D Holden always got word of potential intraoperative disasters. His office suite was adjacent to the bank of operating rooms on the seventh floor of Lakeside Hospital. His grim face and steely blue eyes appeared in the porthole operating room door. We occluded the cava above and below the jagged tear with sponge sticks and ordered our terrified junior residents to exert firm pressure. Tim and I walked away from the table and looked out the window at turbulent Lake Erie, saying little. Only one solution existed, we had to repair this tear. We turned back to the door of the operating suite and reassured Dr. Holden that we had the hemorrhage under control. With the sponge sticks in place, we now extensively and slowly mobilized the large vein, until we could see the rent in its back wall near the spinal vertebral body. We then appreciated adherence between the great vein, the bone and gritty nodules of metastatic pancreatic cancer. A dense inflammatory response had caused our clamp to enter the back of the thin-walled vessel during our dissection. We sutured the rent and completed the caval plication with our back-and-forth silk sutures. This patient's clots were now confined to the legs.

A week later, Dr. Holden called me into the office to discuss the case. He added, "Well, Ralph, if you use heparin properly, you will not have to do that operation very much." Later, Dr. William De Weese devised a serrated clip to partition the cava, a much simpler approach than having to suture the large vein. Minimally invasive, radiological techniques then appeared to place a screen or umbrella within the cava under X-ray guidance. As predicted by Dr. Holden, as we refined our skills with handling anticoagulation, the need for caval interruption decreased. When our medical colleagues pushed for an operation, I transferred potential candidates to surgery, stopped oral anticoagulants, and used precisely monitored doses of intravenous heparin, and often avoided the need for operative intervention. Filters are reserved for patients who cannot receive anticoagulation or when breakthrough embolism occurs in spite of adequate treatment.

Tim and I worked alternate nights during that chief year; neither of us took a vacation. We both wanted see and do as much as possible and, besides this, we were having a great time. That was one of the best years of our lives. We had no neurasthenic concerns about lack of sleep, nor did I ever feel that my abilities were impaired by long hours. I could always sleep the next night. One afternoon, during the spring of chief year, Tim asked me to supervise two of his gallbladder cases the next day as he needed to be away for a day and a half. I asked him the nature of this occasion. He told me that his father had died, and he was attending the funeral in Missouri. He would be back the day after.

Most surgeons are competitive souls. When my staff and I made rounds on Tim's wards, we found that he had admitted two prospective gastric cases and a thyroidectomy to await his return. With the collusion of his junior residents and the patients, we placed bandages and hung fake intravenous infusions. On the morning of Tim's return, we took him on rounds. When he saw his bandaged patients and their intravenous drips, he flushed and his right eye began its lateral migration. We stifled our laughter. Finally, the patients themselves demonstrated the ruse by removing their loosely applied dressings.

Our patients appreciated that residents were truly "their doctors." No utilization review hampered or impeded what we felt was in their best interests. We, also, probably overutilized hospital resources for our own convenience, but we never had to compromise and discharge patients prematurely. Patients' trust had to be earned, but they saw how hard we worked on their behalf. They had faith in our abilities, which gave us faith in ourselves, and, humble as our patients might have been, we clearly grasped what a privilege it was to take care of them as we did. There were no financial incentives, and private practitioners were not involved except when a particular case was difficult enough to demand advanced supervision. But a chief resident had the prerogative to invite an attending to participate. A year after completing my residency, Medicare irrevocably changed surgical education. Financial incentives caused staff services to come under the increased direction and physical participation of attending surgeons so that fees could be collected. Resident responsibility for staff cases gradually eroded, although residents were now provided a living wage. The complexity of the cases also increased, so enhanced senior supervision became, in some cases, a step toward better patient care. Ultimately, financial incentives offered by the program were enough to change the process of surgical education. Medicare is now expensive to taxpayers while, at the same time, failing to provide adequate practitioner compensation. Some practitioners now refuse to accept patients without supplementary insurance. At the same time, questions about quality of care continue to surface. Past analysis of morbidity and mortality outcomes consistently revealed that staff service results by residents were better for patients in major teaching hospitals than in purely private practice hospitals. However, selection of a chief resident was more rigorous than it is now. If a junior resident's performance was inadequate, the director simply let that person go, to find an alternative career. No appeal mechanism existed. Dr. Holden once fired a resident on Christmas Eve for rudeness to a patient. This is no longer true, and residents, even as chiefs, require much supervision.

Upon completing residency at Lakeside Hospital, Tim entered private practice in Missouri and I took up a full-time academic appointment at Western Reserve. Although I elected to spend my life in academics, after all these years, I remember him and admire my surgical colleagues doing general surgery in community settings. The collegiality among fellow residents at Western Reserve contributed to an attitude of mutual respect. My surgical colleagues remained true friends in spite of my quirks and faults, notably impatience, pedantry, and opinions too strongly held. Surgeons are also gentle but careful critics in encouraging my own research efforts. The best of them are open-minded and free of dogmatism.

Internists have unique ways of viewing problems and do not need to be as direct in approaching certain problems as surgeons. This is understandable, given the differences between medical and surgical disease processes. Complicated medical illnesses require time-consuming investigation, while operative interventions are more often needed for processes progressing rapidly or which threaten life or limb. Internists are "customers" of surgeons and we, in turn, need their insights to manage patients in the long term. As a resident, I made regular rounds on the medical floors in the evening. This proactive approach was popular with my medical colleagues because interesting cases often surfaced late in the day. Some required surgical treatment and some did not. This approach avoids late-night or weekend emergency procedures that have high mortality and morbidity.

Cases that do not require surgery are important to consider and to discuss in consultation. One of my encounters on a medical floor provided the basis for a lifetime of personal inquiry into atherosclerosis. A thoughtful senior medical resident called me to see a woman whose serum cholesterol was astronomically high, he thought, because she had a gallstone blocking her bile duct. He knew of my interest in gallstone research and thought that the high blood cholesterol and the gallstone were, in some way, related. I was skeptical of this idea, but I immediately came to examine his patient. Her symptoms were not typical of common duct stone; she had no pain or jaundice, and her gallbladder had been removed. Really, all she had was the biochemical finding of the high serum cholesterol. This resident then produced a contrast study showing a gallstone obstructing a greatly dilated hepatic duct. His thinking was right on the mark. Thirty milliliters of contrast media were worth more than my opinion.

On the day we removed the gallstone, her cholesterol level was 600 mg/dl. As was customary, we left a T-tube in place to drain bile. Two days after the operation, serum cholesterol fell to 140mg/dl and remained at that level the whole time the T-tube functioned. We knew that the bile salts drained from the tube were end products of cholesterol metabolism. As these were excreted from the diverted bile duct, blood cholesterol level fell. Although many, at the time, were skeptical of the lipid hypothesis of atherosclerosis, I believed the evidence that blood cholesterol, in some manner, was related to the development of atherosclerosis. The core of the atheromatous plaque had been demonstrated chemically to consist of esterified cholesterol. In early plaques, as shown by Dr. William Insull Jr., the lipids in the arterial wall were identical to the lipids found in the bloodstream and it appeared that these, most likely, came from the bloodstream. One prominent cardiac surgeon insisted that the artery itself synthesized the lipid within its wall. Others felt that fat was collecting in clots that had formed, and still others felt that blood levels of cholesterol were irrelevant. A way of reducing blood cholesterol levels drastically, I felt, would provide a means of testing the lipid hypothesis.

The Frackleton Foundation of University Hospitals provided funding for initial experiments in dogs that showed that high blood cholesterol levels did cause atherosclerotic plaque formation. We demonstrated that internal biliary diversion could not only prevent but also reverse this process. This was quite exciting. Critics thought that animal models of atherosclerosis were artificial as compared with chronic human disease. However, the plaques in dog arteries appeared to me to be quite similar to those found in humans. Furthermore, these plaques, with time, caused stroke, heart attack, and gangrene in our dogs just as occurred in humans. I regarded biliary diversion as a method to lower blood cholesterol for experimental purposes rather than as a means for treatment. Using serial surgical inspection of opened arteries, we could see that plaques would whiten, shrink and then regress coincident with dramatically lowered cholesterol levels. A consultation from a thoughtful medical resident caused me to spend much of my life thinking about and working on what proved to be a rewarding problem. But clinical challenges tended to divert me from laboratory work.

One such challenge presented itself on the first day of July 1964, as I was beginning my faculty appointment as a junior instructor. A sixty-eight-year-old patient of Dr. Hubay's presented; he was having difficulty swallowing and experiencing upper abdominal pain. Dr. Hubay had just completed a two-stage colon resection for cancer, and had left on a much-needed vacation. The patient's family practitioner had dismissed his swallowing symptoms as a proclivity to abuse alcohol. The patient denied alcohol excess, and I believed him. A contrast study showed cancer involving the lower esophagus and upper stomach. He required an esophagogastrectomy to be done through an extended thoracoabdominal incision. This operation was scheduled within a week of my joining the staff in a junior status. This patient's son was a prominent personal liability attorney in Cleveland, a partner in the firm winning the record Thalidomide judgment. The family, a large and lively mixture of Irish, Italian and Jewish, was well known in the community. The patient, fully aware of my junior status, said that he wanted me to do the operation rather than to wait for my senior partner's return. His attorney son also urged me to go ahead. I got ample advice from junior and senior faculty members not to do this operation. I counseled with Dr. Holden, who asked, "Do you think you can do the procedure?" "Yes, sir." I had done three successfully during my senior year; this was an uncommon procedure. I was as experienced as I needed to be.

I went to church to pray that the faith that the patient and his family had in me be justified. The operation the next day went quite well. Unfortunately, the cancer had spread beyond the confines of the operative field into the lymph nodes, around the diaphragm and the arteries supplying the liver and stomach. It could not be completely removed. However, the patient had eighteen months during which he was relieved of pain and able to eat. The family, aware that we could not remove the entire tumor, was happy to have had this time to share with him. Lessons learned in general practice were useful to me in caring for him during his last days. Liver involvement ultimately caused his death, but he died painlessly in his own bed with his family, priest, and me in attendance.

When John Davis, a pioneer vascular surgeon, became chairman of surgery at the University of Vermont, he left me his practice.

During that first year out of residency, I had done a fair amount of vascular surgery under his direction. However, I felt the need for further experience in this demanding field. Dr. Holden and Dr. Davis arranged for me to spend a month with Dr. Stanley Crawford and Dr. Michael DeBakey in Houston, observing their innovative approaches to arterial surgery. I came away from that institution cognizant of the "Baylor" way, a direct and elegantly simple approach to vascular reconstructions. Dr. Holden did not approve of vacations for his junior faculty; he took none himself. But I stole some time to play poker in Galveston, Texas with my old friend from the air force, Colonel Thomas Lomax Morgan. We relived and remembered some of our happy times in Spain.

A young and well-read neurologist referred the wife of one of our board members for carotid endarterectomy. She had suffered a series of small strokes and retinal damage due to a carotid atheroma, an ulcerated collection of calcium, fat and blood clot at the division of that artery in her neck. Her retinal problem had been misdiagnosed at another prominent center as some type of obscure inflammation. The neurologist had carefully reviewed current literature, documented the attacks, and was struck by the appearance of ocular cholesterol particles. Mr. Rob and Mr. Eastcott in England, and, just prior to that, by Dr. DeBakey, who described his long-term result twenty years later, had done the first carotid endarterectomy less than a decade previously. I had participated in two endarterectomies as a resident, and I had the opportunity to learn the Houston techniques of operative management. I was confident that removing the plaque from an inch or so of carotid artery would not be difficult. However, the surgical procedure was controversial at that time and remained so for many years to come. My immediate problem arose in the form of the professor of neurosurgery. When he saw the case posted on the operative schedule, he called to tell me, "You are doing a case you have no business doing." This message did little to bolster my confidence.

I discussed this gratuitous communication with Dr. Holden, who said, "Tell him to go screw himself." This was a characteristic response from the chief; he could be implacable. I did not repeat his words to the neurosurgeon, a testy man who had pioneered cerebral shunting for hydrocephalus. I respected him, but his abrupt admonition preyed on my nerves. The night before that operation, I went to the racetrack. Winning a few dollars on the daily double was a good omen. We did the operation using local anesthesia, and a junior neurosurgeon was assigned to sit at the head of the table having the patient intone "Methodist Episcopal" every thirty seconds, while continually squeezing a squeaking device with her right hand. In spite the din and the fuss, the procedure was relatively simple and she was quite relieved of her symptoms.

From that time on, I had an excellent referral base for carotid surgery. As techniques evolved, I found that operating under local anesthesia was stressful for the patient, and sometimes even more stressful for me. Often, carotid endarterectomy is a simple and safe operation but, at times, when the plaque extends high into the artery or is adherent and difficult to separate, the procedure can be quite demanding. A small technical defect can cause a devastating stroke. Many papers described methods of performing these operations using electroencephalographic monitoring, general anesthesia and shunts. Some excellent surgeons to this day use local anesthesia and awake monitoring. Techniques for carotid endarterectomy still vary. I encouraged my staff to use the technique that they feel most suitable for the individual patient, and with which they feel most comfortable.

Mistakes also occurred and a lesson I learned from Dr. Alton Ochsner, the senior armed forces consultant in Spain, helped me deal with one serious error. Coincidentally, Dr. Ochsner had been Dr. DeBakey's teacher. Surgery is a small world and these great surgeons had considerable impact on succeeding generations. Dr. Ochsner told us a story about discovering a retained laparotomy tape in a patient after he had done an emergency operation at his clinic. The telltale marker had been spotted on a postoperative radiograph several days after surgery. He immediately informed the patient of this error and removed the tape under local anesthesia through a small strategically placed incision. Within twenty-four hours, an attorney called to solicit a lawsuit while Ochsner's patient was still in the hospital. An underground financially driven network operates in most clinics. Errors do occur and we clearly need to face these head on.

I had operated on an editor of the *Cleveland Press* for a severely compromised leg from an undetected aortic aneurysm. We were able to save a good part of his lower extremity and repaired the aneurysm during his stay. A senior resident closed the abdominal incision. Eighteen months later, the patient appeared in my office with unrelated complaints: an inguinal hernia and a backache. A spine X-ray revealed, in addition to spinal osteoarthritis, a clamp nestled just below the abdominal wall that had been overlooked during closure. A well-intentioned radiologist appeared in my office eager to hand the incriminating pictures to me personally. Remembering Dr. Ochsner's lesson, I immediately showed the films to my patient, illustrating exactly what had happened. I told him that the error was completely my responsibility, adding that the instrument could easily be removed at the time of the hernia repair. On the day of surgery, only my assistant, the patient, and I were aware of the existence of the clamp. After we completed the hernia repair, I made a one-inch incision precisely over the site of the clamp handles and easily removed it. I placed it in sterile gauze, left the operating room, and carried it directly to pathology for cultures. The patient knew that the clamp had been removed through the extra incision. Luckily, there had been no ancillary damage as a result of its presence. He seemed quite content the next morning.

On evening rounds, I found my patient tearful and agitated. During the day, a lawyer had contacted him to tell him that he should sue me. I responded that, indeed, he could, and that he would likely win thirty to forty thousand dollars for the retained instrument. He thanked me and seemed to calm down. I never billed him for the hernia repair. About three months later, in the early spring, I got a call to come to the editor's house on the west side of Cleveland. At that time, I was teaching my two young sons to ride bicycles and I must have mentioned this to him sometime before. I went to his home with a sense of dread. He opened his garage door and produced a vintage Raleigh bicycle that he helped to secure to my car, offering his thanks once again.

While our experimental work continued, the clinical issues of high cholesterol and vascular disease offered a unique opportunity. I saw a fifty-year-old man complaining of calf pain when walking. His serum cholesterol was 350 mg/dl, he was a heavy smoker, and his popliteal artery showed partial occlusion due to plaque. I explained that he might be a candidate for treatment to lower his cholesterol rather than for surgical intervention. He quit smoking completely, followed a cholesterol-reducing diet, and took cholestyramine, a powder that binds bile acids. We checked his progress with serial angiography. As serum cholesterol fell from 350mg to 150mg/dl, two more arteriograms over eighteen months showed that the partial occlusion virtually disappeared. He now walked an unlimited distance without pain.

These angiographic changes correlated with our 1967 animal observations of plaque regression, but we needed much more information to assess the potential arrest, stabilization and possible regression of atherosclerosis in humans. Angiographic images were important, but provided only indirect evidence of improvement in the form of a changing shadow. We could not prove, as skeptics indicated, exactly what had happened within the arterial wall. But I was excited by this finding, and jubilant about the patient's clinical response. This type of clinical observation is anecdotal, but enough anecdotes in the hands of discerning clinicians make data. Case control studies eventually suggested more rigorously designed science and ultimately prospective controlled trials. Years later, coronary and femoral arteriograms documented modest but favorable plaque changes in non-smokers in response to lowered cholesterol along with improved clinical outcomes.

Atherosclerosis was previously considered essentially untreatable and an inevitable consequence of ageing. However, surgical and medical interventions, have evolved to be remarkably effective. Powerful drugs that act on the liver to lower blood cholesterol are now commonly used. While absolute limits of plaque arrest, stabilization, or regression, in response to medical treatment, have yet to be defined, improvements in clinical outcomes in randomized controlled trials are striking. Early partially occluding lesions can be favorably altered and stabilized. The risk of myocardial infarction, stroke and peripheral vascular disease, overall, has decreased coincident with serum cholesterol reduction.

Early in our vascular surgical experience, we recognized that the infection of an arterial graft was a disaster. This problem then caused, and still causes, death or limb loss in about half of patients suffering this complication. After treating four infected aortofemoral bypasses using grafts passed through the obturator canal, we revised our operative and postoperative strategies. On the advice of Dr. Austin Weisberger, then chief of medicine at Western Reserve, we used chloramphenicol and oxacillin, given intravenously immediately preoperatively and for seven days, postoperatively. Chloramphenicol is a feared drug because of the reports of aplastic anemia, particularly when the drug was given orally and to young women. Dr. Weisberger, a hematologist, had taught that chloramphenicol was safe and remarkably effective, provided the drug was given intravenously to adult males or non-menstruating females, rather than orally. He also advocated monitoring of blood counts and a limitation on dosage. Dr. Crawford at Baylor and Mr. Eastcott of St. Mary's in London also advocated using this antibiotic. During the rest of my career, when this regimen was used, there have been only four graft infections in over a thousand cases. Those that did occur related to early discontinuation of antibiotics or failure of the wound to heal. We did not encounter aplastic anemia when chloramphenicol was used with the precautions suggested by Weisberger, nor have I contributed to an extensive literature on graft infection since those first operations for infected grafts.

I advocate intravenous antibiotics with careful monitoring for at least seven days whenever a synthetic graft is placed. My pharmacy colleagues have been most patient, as this recommendation is not "evidence based" because of a relatively low incidence of these disastrous complications. No one would suggest not giving antibiotics and I think the situation is much like that related to ancient debates about the virtues of gloving during surgery. Beyond abnormal lipid metabolism, inflammatory and infectious processes contribute to atherosclerosis, and drugs if they are to be effective, must be given for some period of time.

Our reports on the procedure of obturator bypass proved useful in treating our early groin infections and later, complications related to drug addiction. Most surgeons were more interested in operative technique than in our controversial approach to the prevention of graft infection. A prominent senior surgeon, author of several papers on arterial infections, admonished me for "pickling patients in antibiotics." Antibiotic administration, with known risks, is preferable to the disaster of an infected graft. I had not written about nor had much experience with these infections in my own patients. Overall reported synthetic graft infection rates continue to range about 3-4%, but one graft infection is more than enough to ensure at least amputation and mortality approaching 50%, disastrous prices to pay for current dogmas about limiting antibiotics. I did not have the foresight to do a randomized trial of this course of antibiotic treatment in my vascular patients. I later felt that it would be unethical to do so because of the disastrous consequences of graft infections. Trial data from Scandinavia continues to be published, showing unacceptable infection rates after using one or two doses of antibiotics for a day or two, postoperatively.

One day, a trim gray-haired Italian man appeared in my Lakeside office. He told me he had been advised to have an aortic bypass to remedy severe pain when walking a few feet, and he asked me to perform the surgery. When I asked why he had chosen me, he said he had made inquiries, and believed that I would do a good job. Joseph Di Santa was reputed to be the head of the Mafia in Cleveland. Given his modest demeanor and unassuming appearance, I did not take this information seriously. After arteriograms of his aorta and a check on his heart, which exhibited good contraction although he had documented diffuse coronary disease, he appeared to be a reasonable surgical candidate. He smoked heavily. I asked him to stop smoking and he promised that he would do so.

The morning after the operation, I found two burly guards outside his room. His operation had gone quite well and something else happened. I had begun to perform a type of operation that restored blood flow to the pelvic vessels but spared the genital nerves. Although we had not talked much about this, he again became potent and was possibly more grateful for this, rather than for his ability to walk. On holidays, a large white Cadillac would glide up the driveway to the door of our Cleveland Heights home. The same two large men, Nunzi and Rocco, carried in steaks and bottles of wine for my family. My mother, who was living with us in Cleveland, was distressed by these visits. "If your father knew you had anything to do with those people, he would turn over in his grave."

"Ma, how do I say no to Nunzi and Rocco?"

Joseph also gave University Hospitals cash for an ultrasound scanner that we needed to study aneurysm size. It was hard to dislike him. The prominent urologist who had referred him wanted me to attend meetings of the IAB (Italian American Brotherhood), which were held Wednesday afternoons on Mayfield Road in Cleveland, but I demurred. Everyone who visited the IAB storefront on Murray Hill Road was photographed by the FBI and harassed in one way or another. I had little desire to return to my Italian roots by that route. Joseph had several happy years following his aortic procedure and died later, during coronary surgery. He had wanted to lead a full life, but we had serious disagreements when he appeared in my office deliberately smoking a cigarette. This was an act of overt rebellion. He knew how much this annoyed me and undermined my authority by bringing in trays of pastries and candies, all carried by his henchmen, to bribe our office staff. As far as I was concerned, the office remained a no-smoking zone, and my staff supported my view. We had seen, firsthand, the disastrous effects of continued cigarette smoking on vascular disease.

One night, his wife called my home to tell me that Joseph was having severe chest pain. He had been smoking De Nobili cigars and had consumed a bottle of Lancer's Rose. While I was on my way to see him, a neighboring cardiologist got an electrocardiogram at Joseph's home. This showed a posterior myocardial infarct. We had him admitted to our coronary care unit that night and I chose a particularly strict and personally abstemious cardiologist as his consultant. Joseph had been turned down for coronary bypass before, but this time, the cardiologist who was caring for him got chest pain and had bypass surgery. The cardiologist had a brilliant result with an operation done off pump. He was back making rounds before Joseph left the coronary care unit. Joseph, then, began to lobby for an operation, and, in spite of my reservations, this course was chosen. Unfortunately, he died on the table.

I was told—ordered really—to attend his funeral, which was held at a large funeral home on Mayfield Road in Cleveland Heights. An audience of hundreds was in attendance. He lay in an open casket on white velvet with lilies in his folded hands. As I passed the casket, his wife said, "Doc, there's going to be a lot of trouble. Everybody loved him." I really didn't know how to take this comment. As I was leaving, people were pointing at me, "That's the doctor that operated on him." "No, that's the doctor that did the first operation."

Dark-suited men gathered at the door, studying me carefully though hooded eyes. Then, they walked with me to my car, thanking me for being there and for taking care of their beloved boss. I understood shortly what his wife was talking about. Three cars exploded soon after Joseph's death. One blew up in a bank parking lot near the site of the funeral home, killing an Irishman who was leading a ring to take over the Cleveland organization. Two other cars exploded on the west side of Cleveland as a warning to some dissident Italians.

Part of Joseph's extended family owned an interest in Caesar's Palace. Later, when the University of Nevada was recruiting me as chairman, I traveled with my wife from Cleveland to Las Vegas. I had reservations at the Hilton. A Cadillac picked us up at the Las Vegas airport. Our reservations at the Hilton had been canceled. My wife and I were whisked off to a pink suite at Caesar's Palace with a circular bed on a dais, curtains around it, and a mirror on the ceiling. She scrutinized the bed, and said, "Chief of what?" Whatever might be said, it was their unique way of saying thanks, and it was touching in a hokey way. Las Vegas, glitzy and glamorous, will always be special for me. That night, a married middle-aged couple rode down in the elevator with us. The woman hugged her chubby, bald husband saying, "Thanks for a great time, hon." Las Vegas requires a bit of explanation but, whatever its past history, needs no apology as far as I am concerned.

I wept when I left Cleveland, driving for the last time out of the Mentor Harbor Yacht Club after we won a sailboat race on Lake Erie on a stormy spring day. Dr. Holden had retired, and the new chairman was generous enough to offer me Dr. Holden's named chair. However attractive that prospect might have been, the time had come for me to change course. I tried to convince Dr. Hubay to join me in Reno, Nevada, but he remained rooted in his hometown. As he said, life was never to be easy. Regrettably, the life of that beloved teacher was not easy during his last years. As in sailing or flying, life can mandate 180-degree course changes. I am grateful for compensations of the surgical life and its intensely personal challenges. I wonder, from time to time, what life would have been like had I decided to stay in a comfortable seventh-floor office overlooking Lake Erie. But I am satisfied with the course changes that I made. Though not an easy life as I had been taught in Cleveland, surgery and the move westward unfolded a splendid opportunity. I was not to be disappointed by the new challenges in the Silver State.

RNO-ORD

> Reno sits on a river meadow with her back against the
> High Sierra and her face toward the Great Desert, and
> does not care what people say of her.
> Max Miller

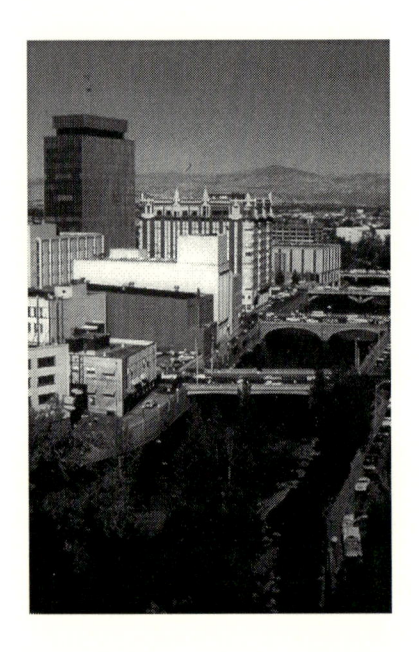

Reno, Nevada in 1979, Courtesy of the
University of Nevada

During the spring and fall of 1979, as I traveled from Cleveland to Reno, my air tickets read RNO-ORD, the last initials signifying the least expensive route via Chicago, as required by the University of Nevada's travel office. Reno, to some of my colleagues, friends, and family, meant gambling, quickie divorces and legalized prostitution. "The Biggest Little City" was described, more accurately in my opinion, as a beautiful woman tucking her skirts up on to the Eastern Sierra slopes and apologizing to no one. But

I had to offer apologies and explanations when I was considering the position of chairman of surgery at a medical school recently founded in the Silver State. My friends and patients in Hunting Valley could not understand why anyone would want to leave Cleveland, "The Best Kept Secret" for the Wild West, and a new medical school founded as a land-grant university, renowned for its school of mines, but even more renowned as a party school.

I knew all this, but the bright light, thin, dry air and the bracing climate of this unique town in the high Northern Nevada desert seemed to energize me, and I got to like the place more and more with each visit. In 1967, the School of Medicine in Nevada had been a gleam in the eyes of Drs. George Smith and Fred Anderson. In 1977, the school converted from a two-year curriculum to a four-year class and Dr. Ernest Mazzaferri from Ohio State was recruited as chief of medicine. He convinced me to accept the position of chief of surgery. Finally, my good friend and patient, Severance Millikan, and Dr. Holden, my chief, sensing my enthusiasm, agreed that this presented a good opportunity.

In spite of propitious prospects for this new school, other colleagues, locally and nationally, disapproved of my choice and of Nevada, in general. Some sneered at Reno as a tired little sin city, notorious for its easy divorces and dude ranches. This was, by far, a highly inaccurate and outdated view. The "Biggest Little City in the World" now had a fine university, a population of responsible citizens who supported the university and its new medical school, and a history in the arts and literature dating back to the turn of the century. While a few community physicians were not eager to see a medical school intrude upon their excellent practices, there was ample support to help launch the teaching effort needed for a four-year school. In spite of my past academic commitment, I understood the viewpoint of the community doctors who were already delivering good care. Many academic medical centers have fine expertise, but some academicians look down on practitioners while living an ivory tower existence, free of call, and shielded from patients by a junior resident staff. Some are talkers, not doers, and cannot be found during evenings and weekends to respond to urgent patient needs. Reno practitioners, mostly U.S. graduates, had committed themselves to their community and their patients twenty-four hours a day, seven days a week. I had seen some of this academic snobbery in an excellent center, but most of my referrals for surgery came from private practitioners in the trenches of patient care and not from full-time medical faculty, who, nonetheless, wished to share in our surgical income. In Reno and in the setting of a new medical school, I felt that we had a unique chance to achieve something quite novel and fine.

Fresh mountain breezes and the pristine gleam of the town, nestled in the Washoe Valley, clear nights with a bright moon rising in the eastern hills, and the forthright demeanor of these Westerners, made this place special. I had been comfortable in my corner office at Lakeside Hospital in Cleveland, probably too comfortable. And I was becoming bored. I looked out each day over the dull green waters of Lake Erie. I had sailed the length and breadth of our inland sea and knew it, and its moods, intimately. I also knew, were I to stay where I was, that little would change. I would not be a candidate for the chair at Case Western Reserve, nor would any surgeons trained by Dr. William D Holden be chosen. The dean wanted candidates not associated with the traditions of our department and his search committee appeared to agree. I came to learn that these attitudes are common when new chairs are recruited. An outside candidate is seen as a "white knight," in spite of the achievements of the members of the incumbent department. This happens in corporate recruiting as well, but academic politics can be even more petty and vicious, some say, because the stakes are picayune.

So I journeyed RNO-ORD with members of my laboratory staff and my secretary from Cleveland to negotiate the shape of what would become the Department of Surgery at the University of Nevada School of Medicine. A distinguished professor in the English department of the University of Nevada, Reno, a patient and later, a friend, had told me, "A move to Reno might seem to be a chancy and parlous undertaking." But he, a discerning literate man, loved the place and had raised a fine family there. During a preliminary interview with Dr. Robert Gorrell, then vice president of academic affairs, I received a subtle quiz about Chaucer. I enjoyed meeting Dr. Gorrell, and decided to take the job. I guessed that I had passed his quiz. Over the years, I also came to admire the soft-spoken president, Dr. Joseph Crowley, "The Velvet Hammer", a political scientist and strong supporter of the new medical school. He guided UNR's spectacular growth over the next two decades.

My two periods of service at The University of Nevada School of Medicine proved to be important and productive periods in my professional life. Initially, John Wilburn, our skilled laboratory assistant, decided to join me in my move to Reno. We packed our large laboratory at Case Western Reserve. He supervised the safe transfer of our precious colony of atherosclerotic dogs and monkeys to the veterinary school at the University of California at Davis, as no animal facilities existed in Reno that time. Dean Fred Robbins at Case Western Reserve generously gave me permission, as principal investigator, to move our laboratory equipment, including much needed ultracentrifuges and an RCA EMU-3G electron microscope to new laboratories at the medical school just north of town.

Dr. Ernest Mazzaferri, the chair of medicine, from Ohio State, was an outstanding teacher and clinician. He radiated unbridled enthusiasm for medicine and all things connected with the care of the sick. Dr. Thomas Scully, a pediatrician, tall and silver-haired, appeared to be the best-looking dean in American medicine. He came originally from New Rochelle, New York, and had been attracted to the high desert of Nevada after serving as an air force doctor in Spain. He left his duties due to illness shortly after I arrived, and had been a pleasure to work with. He facilitated the school's transition from a two—

to a four-year curriculum. Dr. Mazzaferri then served as acting dean. While I was being recruited, I met Dr. Malcolm Edmiston, a local surgeon who had been the acting surgical chair. He was a spare tan gentleman clad in Western garb, long slender trousers and trim jackets with gussets and leather buttons. On my third visit, he suggested that I host a Reno Surgical Society meeting. We arranged this event at Vario's, fine restaurant on Virginia Street. Twenty-nine of the local surgeons came, and after a liberal cocktail hour and a series of outrageous jokes, they began to ask questions. Beating around the bush was not their style. They wanted to know what I intended to do and what I expected of them. I outlined the medical student program emphasizing broad exposure to general surgery and a residency program based both in Las Vegas and Reno. The prospect of resident assignments in Reno made them grumble. In contrast to surgeons back East, they did not want or need residents to do "scutwork" or to take their night calls. They managed their own workups, as well as pre—and postoperative care, and, as I was soon to learn, they were doing an excellent job.

Particular senior surgeons, Dr. Kenneth Maclean, Dr. Fred Anderson, the Cantelon brothers and the neurosurgeon, Dr. Ernest Mack, had long before set a high and ethical standard for the practice of surgery. These men, superbly trained and highly motivated, supported the school's development, but placing residents in private hospitals in Reno remained a highly charged issue for most of the younger surgeons. Dr. Maclean interviewed candidates applying for the Nevada Licensing Board. He had a way of asking questions on the oral examination, which would ferret out weak candidates.

We sat around the big table at Vario's and, after dessert, their feelings and attitudes became clear. They appeared to like me but distrusted the persona of a new medical school. I appreciated their directness and frank expression of opinion, whether pro or con; this was something rarely seen back East. After dinner, the headwaiter handed me a bill for $1,572. I could see "my guests" looking at me covertly, with poker eyes and closely held expressions. I paid the bill without comment, using my American Express card. As we strolled to the parking lot, I glanced at Dr. Edmiston, and without prompting, he commented, "You are now a member of the Reno Surgical Society."

"And what does that mean?" I asked.

"Well, each of us takes a turn at hosting. They liked you, so you are now a member of the Reno Surgical Society. You will get free dinners for the next thirty months, and you will hear some good jokes."

Later, I met members of the American College of Surgeons who had heard that it cost $1,500 to become a member of the Reno Surgical. In a way, this was true; this was about the price of one of the "hosted" dinners. My initial investment in the Reno Surgical Society dinner was worth every cent. Each host tried to outdo the next by arranging dinner meetings in outstanding places. I looked forward to monthly dinner meetings and the fellowship of that group. Two surgeons, each on call, were not allowed to drink whatsoever. These on-call martyrs were pitied and fussed over. Sharp-eyed patrolmen regularly appeared outside restaurants hosting the event to make certain that everyone got home safely. Nevada police officers, unfailingly polite, could be quite severe. They also knew most of the doctors in town by name, and DUI was a serious offense. My car still had Ohio license plates six weeks after my arrival. One night, a policeman rang my bell at 746 Marsh to remind me that I was now a Nevadan and that I should have Nevada license plates.

One of the hosted meetings of the Reno Surgical months later convened in a colorful place on 4th Street in Sparks called the Coney Island Bar and Grill. The place was famous for ample Wednesday night family-style dinners, but was definitely not a gourmet establishment. At the time, sawdust graced the floor and a sign over the bar read, "Cowboys must remove shit from their boots before entering." Dinner consisted of pitchers of beer, hot dogs, sauerkraut, and fried chicken. At the end of the usual round of jokes, and after a bewildered speaker presented his lecture, the host, a distinguished specialty surgeon, rose. He asked, "You might wonder why you are all here." "To tell the truth," someone replied, "we were wondering why you chose this place and this type of meal." At that moment, three minivans pulled up to the Coney Island B&G. Their destination was to be the Mustang Ranch, a licensed brothel. Our host told us that drinks only, not other favors of the house, were to be at his expense.

This was an opportunity to see firsthand one of the most fabled whorehouses in Nevada. Joe Comforte's famous ranch lay a few miles east of town in Storey County off of Route 80. The structure consisted of trailers and low-lying buildings all knit together in a kind of trailer park configuration. A fence surrounded the rambling structure and a dirt road ran directly to a sturdy iron gate, which admitted our vehicles to an empty parking lot. As the group approached the front door, a loud bell clanged three times. Double doors were flung open and about twenty good-looking, well-dressed women formed a semicircle to greet us. All we were required to do was to look them over and they, laughing, looked back at us. Then, the line of ladies dispersed. Some went to the bar, some to tables, and others, to parts unknown. They had quickly sized us up as a bunch of non-swingers. Doctors, the bartender later told me, were notoriously cheap. The house preferred truck drivers.

According to stories told and later retold, all the members of our party had after-dinner drinks, and that was it. All hands were accounted for when the minibuses went back to 4th Street. Prostitution was legal in the state of Nevada, and these nice, clean-cut young women looked like junior versions of Kitty out of *Gun Smoke*. I was surprised at how attractive and personable they were. I commented on this to an older well made-up lady who seemed to be in charge. She looked me square in the eyes, replying with a broad smile, "Sure, who would pay to screw an ugly girl?" I fantasized that that was the experience of the true old West, rather than the reality of a recreational stop for tired truck drivers halfway between Winnemucca and San Francisco. Even so, there was a good-natured openness about the place. I later thought that the madam had not been exactly right; I have seen men that have paid dearly for consorting with ugly women. This night was eventually recognized, depending on one's point of view, as a zenith or nadir of the Society's activities. The Reno Surgical now has a diverse membership, with biannual meetings attended by more than 100 guests, wives and students. Guest lecturers, who come once a year, are sometimes stuffy and sometimes quite refreshing. For example, Judge Mills Lane on Nevada gun control, "This means two hands on the gun." Nevada has always tolerated and cherished personal freedom. Most women born there love their state and defend it. In contrast, some Eastern women, sight unseen, despise Nevada. At a dinner party with a distinguished judge, our dean's wife complained about legalized prostitution and establishments such as the Mustang and the Chicken Ranch in the south. The judge's wife set her straight, "The Mustang is every Western man's right. When we came here in covered wagons, few women would come."

Her husband then added, "The houses are legal, Doc, but if you move a girl into your house, we will know about it tomorrow on Court Street."

Old Reno had the patina of a man's place, but, then, no pornographic films were exhibited in Washoe County in contrast to Times Square or downtown Cleveland. Current newspaper publicity either deplores or sensationalizes the old houses. Either way, the discussion will presage the end of an era. But then, the prevalence of AIDS in Nevada brothels is virtually zero. The law requires weekly checkups and safe sex.

Before I left Cleveland, I spent a few days skiing in the Sierra with my son Ted to consider his senior year at University School in Cleveland. I put the question to him on the ski lift in Heavenly Valley, indicating that leaving would be a sacrifice for him. As I recall, Ted quickly replied, "Sure, okay." This was the decision I needed. Recently he told me that he had really said, "Surely you jest!" But he did go back to Cleveland to graduate with his high school class. Interestingly, compared to Cleveland, he still regards the pretty little city on the edge of the Sierra as small-town USA.

I began my tenure on April Fool's Day in 1980. That spring, I had been wearing a fur hat in the still frigid Cleveland weather, and I was capped in fur as I walked down the long Quonset hut that served as our airport structure. Dr. Mazzaferri, squinting at me down the 50-yard length of the ramshackle corridor, appeared anxious. As I drew closer and removed the fur hat, he seemed relieved. "My God, Ralph, I thought it was a wig. Anyone who came to Reno might be crazy." We agreed that most men who might wear wigs might be a bit crazy and on many other things as well. I once took care of Frank Sinatra's wig maker, who insisted that I visit him for a fitting. I was bald as a young man during residency. The wig maker and his wife wanted to make me a present of a wig and I had to fight them off. They finally gave me a nice robe for my wife, but I could see that they really wanted me to have a hairpiece. I dread to think of the reaction of my fellow surgical residents had I appeared in a toupee. I now prefer a partially shaved head.

We immediately began caring for veterans at the Ioannis A. Lougaris Veterans Medical Center. The students accompanied us during rounds on private patients at St. Mary's and Washoe. The Veteran's Administration's director, Harry Potter, and the chief of staff, Dr. Paul Jensen, welcomed the new medical school's educational efforts. Later, Dr. Richard Bomberger and Dr. Byron McGregor joined Dr. Robert Merchant in staffing our teaching service. The students were interesting. While they appeared as laid-back informal young people, they were, in a way, more highly motivated and energetic than typical Eastern students. They could hardly wait to get to work in the morning. Accustomed to rising early, one group with rumbling trucks and banks of headlights appeared at my house before dawn so we could start rounds even earlier than I might have wished. Some took me into the desert to demonstrate the capabilities of their four-wheeled vehicles. Their enthusiasm was contagious. Most students were Nevadans; a few hailed from Alaska, Idaho and Montana. The "sage brush stamp" and high grades were required for admission and these young people were a minority of sorts.

Before the medical school was founded, only three or four young Nevadans were accepted to "out-of-state" medical schools. The traditional academic establishment had not been kind to young people from the Silver State in terms of medical school admissions. Each class at the new Nevada Medical School seemed to have a unique character. The class of 1982 was able to party all night, get up early and still do a day's work. They were avaricious for medical knowledge and soaked up everything that the faculty could dish out. Some of the best students would read the latest journals to then challenge the faculty on morning rounds. When they did this, it was wise to get up early or to run for cover.

Mormon students, who were among my first group, in the class of 1980, were unusually serious and reserved. My first group of student clerks, gathering at the Marsh Street cottage, was served beer, Coca-Cola, pretzels, and pizza. My housekeeper, Marie Shultz, whispered to me that none of them were touching the beverages. She told me they were "LDS," standing for Latter Day Saints, the preferred term. I had not encountered LDS students and did not know that they did not use alcohol, drink caffeinated beverages or eat chocolate. Marie dashed down California Avenue to the supermarket for Seven-Up and ginger ale. These students, all married, had grave-looking young wives, who clustered around Marie, engaging her in a serious conversation.

The women had noticed that I was living alone in the thatched cottage on Marsh Avenue. The next night, I returned home to a beautifully set table and a casserole in the oven. This went on for several nights. Thinking that Marie, the housekeeper, was cooking my dinner, I called her at home to thank her. She explained that the students' wives believed that men should be taken care of and asked for a key. In other words, I was to be fed in the spirit of family values traditional among LDS wives. But this was too generous and really too much to ask of anyone, particularly from someone not planning a conversion to their faith. But the casseroles were not bad while they lasted. Duplicitously, I had Marie tell the wives that Italians eat special food.

The house at 746 Marsh Street was most unusual in many

ways. Photographs of it have graced architectural magazines nationally. Dean Scully had found it for me and arranged a lease with option to purchase. The house had been built by an architect as a model of a French cottage where he and his wife honeymooned somewhere in the south of France. The cottage had cut, cast-leaded windows, beams and a real thatched roof. Because I thought I might have to move to Las Vegas, I leased the house.

The house was haunted. The first night that I arrived in Reno, arrangements had been made for me to stay at the MGM Grand. Instead, I went the house and I saw that my car was in the cottage driveway. I opened the door to let my Siamese cat, Mali Ying, out of her carrying case. She explored the place and appeared to approve of it, and quickly curled upon a United Airlines blanket, a gift from the flight attendants on that final flight West. I found that the housekeeper had set up my bed and that the movers had placed the furniture in some semblance of order, so I ate out and came directly home. Affected by a three-hour time difference, I was asleep as soon as I got into bed. The phone rang. The manager of the MGM said that he had been expecting me: he was calling to be sure I was okay. I assured him that I was and was instantly asleep once more.

At about one o'clock, I was abruptly awakened once again by the distinct sound of footsteps on creaky wooden floors. Mali Ying, at the foot of the bed, arched her back and growled. Siamese cats, once temple guardians, do this in times of peril, and they are quite vocal. Her loud yowling and dramatic posturing got my attention, and I sat bolt upright. Groaning, I loaded my shotgun, got a flashlight and cautiously stalked the place. There was nothing but a howling northwest wind, Mark Twain's "Washoe Zephyr," and the house seemed quite cold for April. But the wind did not account for the footsteps or my cat's reaction. The casement windows and outside doors were securely locked. I searched the closets and checked the room over the garage and its hallway and found nothing. A tour of the grounds yielded nothing but howling Sierra winds and rustling garden shrubs. The noise stopped, and I crawled, shivering, back into bed. Mali Ying insisted on joining me under the covers. Recurrent disturbances continued while I lived there. These seemed to start at about 1 to 2 in the morning, and I noticed that they occured when the house was messy. The specter, a silent older woman, finally appeared one night in June. I could not make out her features, but I was struck by a feeling of deep sadness. I had, once again, been awakened from a sound sleep, and Mali Ying was doing her alarm growls and back arches, so this was no dream. She appeared at the bedroom door on my right, looking in at me. Turning to the door, I shouted, "Don't worry, we will take care of your house."

She made no reply, but after my loud shout, it became quieter for some weeks. For several reasons, I became convinced that the phenomenon that I experienced was real. Many "Old Reno" residents still talk about the fact that 746 Marsh is haunted. I later learned that, within the last decade, priests from Our Lady of Snows had performed an exorcism there. I would feel uncomfortable in telling this story, had it not been that others had heard and seen her as well. Ten days after my arrival, I had an abrupt phone call from someone asking me to appear and give a lecture in London at the Charing Cross Vascular Symposium. Somehow, during the move, this invitation had been lost in the mail. A week later, on my return from London, Dr. Mazzaferri was on hand at the airport Quonset hut to greet me with another worried look and a story of "Trouble on Marsh Street." On short notice, two medical students had kindly agreed to care for the house and Mali Ying. One young woman was to sleep there but she got frightened at one o'clock in the morning. She called her boyfriend to stay over the next night. After two nights' experiences with footsteps, they both fled to return only in the daytime to feed the cat. They were certain that someone was in the house each night. The two students thought that someone had gotten in through the windows, though all of them were locked.

I became busier and slept soundly during the cool dry nights and I had no time to worry about ghosts. I later learned that the woman for whom the house had been built had suffered sudden sharp abdominal pain at midnight and was taken to St. Mary's Hospital. Dr. Maclean had operated for acute diverticulitis and, quite unexpectedly, she died on the table at about one in the morning. The surgeon could never understand why this happened. He related the history sadly and haltingly, saying that he had never come to a closure with this event. Coincidentally, Dr. Maclean himself later died during surgery at that same hospital.

Some of my patients came from Cleveland and Cincinnati for vascular procedures in Reno, and these went quite well. I also kept busy scrubbing with the local Reno surgeons, who were proctoring my surgery, as was done for any new surgeon coming to town. It was fun to work with accomplished operators from various programs and we learned from each other. I worked on vascular cases at the VA with Bob Merchant, and did general surgery with Malcolm Edmiston in town. Dr. H. Treat Cafferata, educated at Stanford and trained at UCSF, was most supportive and we eventually published some technical innovations. His direct manner kept me from having to operate upon unreasonable cases referred by a full-time medical colleague. Mrs. Kathleen Lewis came to supervise our office, shepherding patients and helping set up a corporate practice on a sound financial basis.

My associates and I took calls in each of the two emergency rooms, offering to give up our calls, at anytime, for local surgeons desiring work. This had been a problem, as the former surgical appointee was perceived as taking more than his fair share of cases from the emergency rooms. The operating room nurses at all the facilities were remarkably competent. They were old-fashioned classic operating room nurses who understood surgical procedures and anticipated each new step. Although some local surgeons were dubious about the need for a medical school in Nevada, they were thoughtful in helping me schedule cases and in seeing that the assistance I got in the operating room was the best. Anesthesia was outstanding, with minimum fuss compared to the usual university mess of a fumbling advanced resident brigade. An excellent Persian anesthesiologist in Cleveland, Dr. Ali Gharib, recommended Dr. Massoud Dorostkar, also Persian and practicing in Reno. Ali Garib always got into the OR first in Cleveland and got the cases going with a smooth uneventful anesthetic. Dr. Dorostkar's modus operandi was exactly the same. Massoud, in contrast to the other local anesthesiologists, would not hesitate to do the many charity cases the university service in Reno attracted. When I once asked him why, he said, "This country gave me much. I am giving it back."

Our application for surgical residency training at the Reno VA Medical Center and Southern Nevada Memorial Hospital in Las Vegas was approved to begin in 1981. One of my former students, Dr. Charles Buerk, came as vice chairman to supervise the program in Las Vegas. Dr. Buerk had always been interested in burns, and he and Dr. John Batdorf developed a burn center in Las Vegas that became a premiere facility with a fine trauma center as well. It took a while for me to finally settle in Reno because Las Vegas wanted and needed surgical residents while the surgical community in Reno wanted to do without them except at the Veterans Hospital. Hospital hunting for the residency site in Las Vegas became a novel adventure. I visited a large hospital, famous for its coronary care unit, which was the size of a football field. The unit was always full of male victims of gambling excitement or other Las Vegas indulgences. The coronary care unit had made the newspapers because the nurses had been found to be, or at least were suspected of, taking bets on who would live or die. Thus, the legend of "Angels of Death" circulated in the local press. The rumor was unfair; this hospital was excellent. But my review of surgical caseload determined that insufficient variety existed to support a general surgical training program.

The hospital administrators in Las Vegas were unusual as compared to conservative managers I had worked with in the past. When traveling, I wore three-piece dark suits, just as my Cleveland mentor, Dr. Holden, had done. I once asked the chief why he always wore dark suits. He said that he did not have to worry about the color of his stockings. Dealing with businessmen with plunging necklines and medals on gold chains peaking out of gray-haired chests was unsettling. But in spite of appearances, these were competent and helpful people who knew exactly what they needed. In Las Vegas, they wanted the University Services to work at their hospitals and were willing to back this desire by supporting resident salaries. Because of its trauma work and a fine cardiac surgery program headed by a surgeon trained by Dr. Michael DeBakey, the final choice of our hospital for resident education was the Southern Nevada Memorial Hospital, now called University Hospital.

Mr. George Reisz, an administrator at SNMH, welcomed our first surgical residents to Las Vegas, who were sent by Dr. Jeffrey Ponsky, a former Lakeside resident, then chief of surgery at Mt. Sinai Hospital in Cleveland. The Cleveland residents were delighted with this rotation, confirming the correctness of that venue for our training program in Las Vegas. I vacillated on where to live, finally deciding on Reno because of the need for laboratory facilities for research and interactions with the basic scientists at the Reno campus. I commuted to Las Vegas every two weeks to conduct mortality and morbidity conferences.

Las Vegas is quite distinct from the rest of the Silver State, which is essentially rural, with wide, open spaces and ranches and mines and small towns. This is a big city, with big shows, big crowds and great excitement. Las Vegas is, in fact, like no other place in the world. The *New Yorker* praised the town as a paradigm of a vibrant city. It gave a kind of qualified praise, mostly because of crowds of people, many of them walking. Visitors will not see the Metropolitan Museum but they can scrutinize an art collection at the Bellagio, enjoy the marvels of mega hotel casino architecture, and dine well and more conveniently than in New York. Instead of mobbed New York museums, the Bellagio exhibition in Las Vegas can be easily viewed at ten dollars per head and no fuss. The best Las Vegas restaurants, such as the Napa, rival those of London, New York, and even Paris. The *New Yorker* struggled to describe this unique place, but made of it something more than it really is. Other writers have depicted Las Vegas as a paradigm of evil, which recently elected a "mob lawyer" as mayor, an unfair accusation.

Las Vegas is an exquisite playground, initially catering to adults, and now attracting families. It is the most spectacular destination resort in the world. First-generation Italians and Jews created this fantasyland, and there is no other place like it. Benjamin Seigel gave his life for it, and Moe Dalitz and Meyer Lansky supported the improbable idea of a destination resort in the middle of a barren desert. Gaming and shows are the main things but the spirit of the West and the openness and energy of the Silver State made this dream possible, along with a brilliant engineering feat, the Hoover Dam, which supplies the power needed for all that flamboyant lighting. The phenomenon might happen elsewhere, but I doubt that it will. Atlantic City, which appears gray, sullen and nasty, will never compete with Las Vegas, unless New Jersey miraculously imports the generous Western spirit. There is something else. The freedom to sin, to lose or to win is the exact opposite of prescribed Eastern strictures. These freedoms are also the exact opposite of what radical Islam, our new enemy, wants to force upon us and the rest of the world. Las Vegas is what it is and I love it. In a flashback, I saw myself at a site visit for a research grant at the University of Iowa, asking, "Can a medical school like the one in Nevada actually work?"

Sandra Daugherty, M.D., Ph.D., the epidemiologist assigned to the project replied, "It can and my husband is the one who can make it work."

Dr. Robert Daugherty succeeded brilliantly in Nevada. Before Daugherty was recruited, it was suggested that Dr. Mazzaferri or I consider the dean's position. But Dr. Mazzaferri wanted to be chief of medicine and I wanted to do surgery. The search for a dean was agonizing and protracted, and unlikely people, including a "cardiovascular surgeon," an assistant dean in Washington, D.C., who flew in and out in one day after meeting briefly with the local physicians, offered the opinion that a medical school in Nevada would never work. He was wrong, of course.

Dr. Robert Daugherty, with considerable energy and a mandatory degree of ruthlessness, built the school on a foundation already established by an able administrative staff. Bob, a tall, good-looking man from Kansas, was the son of a general practitioner. He believed in the "generalist initiative" and the need for rural medicine in the state. Dr. Mazzaferri and I, as specialists, did not agree with him on certain issues, but he respected and supported research efforts and dedication to specialty practice as long as our students received a broad education. He was hardworking and energetic. We set up conferences for local physicians and toured the whole state in a van, all the chiefs, with Bob driving so fast some of us had white knuckles. We met doctors in little towns like Battle Mountain, Fernley, Tonopah and Winemucca and Ely, and in a "big town" like Elko. Practitioners were often interested in the latest antibiotics to take care of the local working girls; the general surgeons were interested in the latest advances in shock and trauma. Dr. Mazzaferri lectured on thyroid disease, as an epidemic of thyroid cancer and adenomas in Southern Nevada also extended to the North as well as into Utah. We thought that these tumors might relate to the radioactive fall out in the late '40s and early '50s, but the federal government did not think much of our idea of a grant to investigate the legacy of atomic testing in Nevada.

We were insanely busy, and I loved every minute of it. My Tartan 33-foot sloop, *Artemis II*, now plied beautiful blue Tahoe instead of green Lake Erie and was crewed by Nevada medical students, mostly desert rats. But one student, Pendleton Alexander, class of 1982, was a competitive Finn sailor from southern California who proved to be a leader. He is now chief of cardiothoracic surgery at the Washington D.C. Veterans Hospital, which, from time to time, had to suspend cardiac surgery before his arrival. We collected our trophies for weekend regattas and, on one memorable Fourth of July, we finished first overall in the Trans-Tahoe race.

When residents arrived in 1981, the educational program accelerated in a gratifying way. But then, I received a call in late 1982. The search committee for chair of surgery at George Washington School of Medicine wanted me to consider that position. The invitation came during a visit from good friends from Chicago, Dr. John Bergan and his wife Elisabeth, who kidded me about my happiness in "Reno Nirvana." My wife, daughters and mother-in-law were also overjoyed at the prospect of a move to Washington, which appeared to offer more educational opportunities for our two daughters. I was also flattered. This did seem to be a promising opportunity. The George Washington Hospital was three blocks from the White House and their trauma service had saved President Reagan after a gunshot wound.

I anticipated a chance to help create a great clinic and educational center in the nation's capital city. But accountants, who managed our straightforward university surgeons' practice plan, looked over financial statements sent by the administration at George Washington Hospital. The balance sheet was totally incomprehensible, and Kafoury Armstrong, an excellent accounting firm in Reno, told me that they could not interpret the statement. I paid $500 for this opinion, which later proved to be essentially correct. I later found out that the surgical department had suffered chronic financial losses, not evident from the accounting provided, and that other departments had to chip in to cover bonuses already paid to faculty members. Just before I left, another ominous note sounded. I had recruited an intern from George Washington's Medical School. He was disappointed that I was relinquishing my Nevada post. I learned from him that the residency program was not only on probation, but had been formally disapproved. He said, "Don't go to that terrible place."

He wrote on my going-away card, "You have tiger by the tail."

I have learned to always listen to what residents have to say. Unfortunately, he was correct. This move gave me some fine challenges but also some of the most miserable times in my life. Misery began with having to write and reorganize a residency program that was a true disaster. The assistant "cardiovascular" dean, the same one who had visited our school in Nevada, had told me that this was a matter easily corrected with a little paperwork. This was, at worst, a lie and, at best, a serious misjudgment. But the prospect of Washington, D.C., seemed heady at the time, so I overlooked the obvious warning signs.

After twelve years, I returned to the Silver State in 1993, not having done as much as I had hoped in Washington, D.C. At one point, I nominated Joseph Crowley for the presidency of George Washington University and got a letter politely declining this candidacy. Washington is an unusual city. According to dramatic headlines in the *Washington Post*—and all of their headlines are dramatic—the city could be viewed as a culture literally eating itself alive. Monika Lewinsky, in addition to being terrorized by the FBI for eighteen hours in a hotel room, was required to testify before a grand jury. President Clinton had lied about questions that, in my opinion, no one should have asked in the first place. Reflecting on sexual mores and Nevada traditions, I think that, had William Jefferson Clinton patronized the Mustang Ranch for a bit of fellatio, this would have been perfectly legal. It might not have been as anonymous as one might wish. The girls kept track of who came to see them, and somehow, they liked to brag about celebrities. I know a prominent citizen, a regular patron, who dressed in old clothing and represented himself as a truck driver, because, according to him, the girls then charged less. The cost differential in Clinton's case might have been fifty or seventy-five dollars, as opposed to fifty million of our taxpayer dollars, to support the activities of Kenneth Starr and associates, and the outcome would likely have been better for our country. Easterners view Nevada with snickering disapproval, but I am convinced that the Nevada approach to such matters is straightforward and honest.

On my return to Nevada in 1994, I was refreshed by the cool breezes of our afternoon "Washoe Zephyr" and relieved to escape the heat and humidity of Washington. When I slept, the bed remained barely disturbed. Arising on winter and spring mornings, I saw snow on Mount Rose and the gleaming little town in the valley below. The population of Nevadans had grown from seven hundred thousand in 1980 to about 1.5 million by that time. The school graduated fine classes of students who competed well for excellent residencies. I am confident that those that follow will be just as good.

People in the West sometimes use the words "back East" with a deferential tone. They do this with a sense of respect for all that past history. For all its culture and sophistication, I still see it as "backward East," plagued with more than its rightful share of hang-ups, hostilities and snobbery. The nightmarish quality of problems in Washington became hard to envision in the bright lights of

Nevada. I laughed a lot driving down the foothills each morning to our new veterans hospital, now called the VA Sierra Nevada Health Care Network. There are always problems to solve in this complicated time for medicine, but somehow, these seemed a bit easier in a setting of optimism and honesty. Sometimes, gritty straight talk makes all the difference.

The state of Nevada continues to graduate class after class of fine young doctors with sagebrush stamp, and I am proud to have had a part in that. But then, another challenge appeared. A course change at the turn of the century would once again take me back to Washington as national director of surgery for the Department of Veterans Affairs. Neither Robert Gorrell nor Joe Crowley was happy when I discussed it with them. They told me, "You have already tried that." The ever-enthusiastic neurosurgeon, Dr. Ernest Mack encouraged me to accept the position. It remains to be seen how this new challenge will turn out.

WASHINGTON YEARS: HIGH HOPES AND PARTISAN POLITICS

Washington, this inadvertent Rome
This Goetheless Weimar
This Samarkand of kinless desperadoes
Charles McCarry

Perhaps even this will someday give us pleasure to remember
Aeneas, Virgil

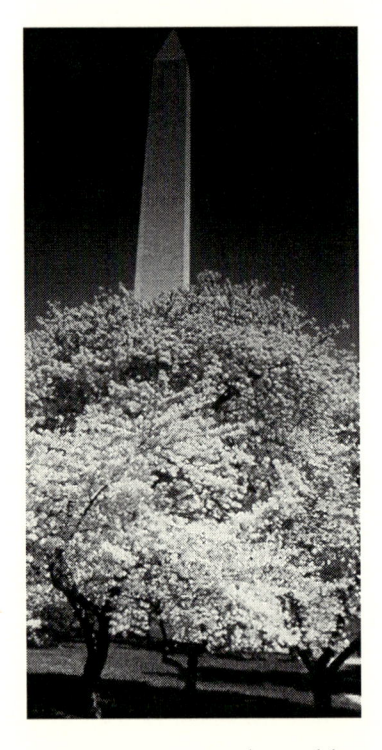

Washington Monument in cherry blossom time

Once I accepted the chair at George Washington University, my family left Three Newlands Circle in Reno to arrive in Washington in time for our daughters, Lee and Mindy, to begin the school year in September. My laboratory assistant, John Wilburn, and I followed, driving across the country in a new 1982 Diesel Mercedes. Such were sensitivities in academic medicine that Dr. Mazzaferri, chief of medicine, and I had both purchased similar cars that we deemed sufficiently modest for academicians. The Mercedes carried my more valuable artwork and our laboratory records. Jesus Cortez, "Chucho," an earnest young Mexican, who worked for a local judge, also volunteered to come. At the last minute, although he had a visa, he changed his mind, fearing that Washington, D.C., might itself be the "*gran migra*," as Latinos referred to our immigration service. Although he was a legal immigrant, he still feared that, in some way, he might be sent back to Mexico. These fears were unfounded. Actually, immigration enforcement was much tougher in Nevada than on the East Coast. Chucho remained behind looking after the big house at Three Newlands, continuing his education, and ultimately becoming a United States citizen. We were fortunate because the house took a long time to sell, and Chucho continued as a caretaker. I went back twice to Reno, and as we walked the grounds, we both wept, recalling our fine parties with medical students and newly recruited surgical residents.

Early on the morning we left, just east of Reno on Route 80, we passed a hodgepodge of buildings to the right of the highway and on the Truckee riverbank. This was the complex of the Mustang Ranch bordello. I commented, "Well, John, that's the last time we'll ever see that." He bridled, "Well, they don't let us in there, anyway." Until that moment, I had not known about that policy of the Mustang Ranch toward people of color. John's sudden anger surprised me; ordinarily an amiable companion, John reminded me of my old friends in the Bronx. We had a tradition of attending Cleveland Indian baseball games with our sons, and I looked forward to this seven-day drive with him so we could see some of our great country. One of the

Nevada medical students had raved about the grandeur of a cross-country automobile journey. He proved quite correct. We encountered only a little bit of unpleasantness. Stopping at a bar for lunch somewhere in the middle Wyoming on our second day, several tough-looking cowboys and a grizzled bartender turned to glare at us as we entered. Sensing their overt hostility, I felt that I had to say something. Grinning, I said lightheartedly, "Well, here is trouble if you are looking for it." John stood 6'6" and weighed 290 pounds. He stood beside me, glowering. The bartender looked down and the cowboys turned their attention to their beers. A skinny waitress, her sun-damaged skin wrinkled in smiles, served us rare hamburgers. We ate quickly and silently then continued our journey East on Route 80.

Upon crossing the Great Divide, the landscape abruptly turned from the dun tan of the West to dark green. After a fine steak dinner in Omaha, we stayed in the same pleasant roadhouse for the night. The next afternoon, in Iowa, on a whim, we turned off the great highway and drove twenty-five miles north on a secondary road to a small farm town where a lively baseball game was in progress. Hefty-looking men and women in bib overalls invited us to the home team dinner. They seemed pleased to have us there, so we stayed for two days, rooting for the hometown team, which won the little series. We pressed eastward through Chicago, arriving in Cleveland by nightfall. John visited his family on the East side and I stayed with an old friend, Greta Milliken, at Ripplestone in Hunting Valley for a day of rest, a fine meal, and good conversation with that great lady. She chided me for having gained weight. After an easy drive from Cleveland, we came, by late afternoon, to Bethesda, Maryland, where Eve had rented a home. The bill for diesel fuel totaled seventy-six dollars. This Mercedes turbo diesel, though far from glamorous, had been a good investment. But our temporary home was not at all as fine as Three Newlands Circle and I already missed my home in the Silver State.

Early the next morning, we drove down Canal Road into the District of Columbia. Although September can be a fine month in Washington, that day was hot and humid, and the kudzu overhanging the canal road gave us a feeling of driving into a swamp. After wide, open Western spaces, the congested district traffic and the crowded parking in the George Washington Medical Faculty Associates building were unsettling. We had negotiated a position for John in the Surgical Laboratories as chief technician, with a six thousand-dollar raise guaranteed over his University of Nevada salary. As we unloaded books and research records into dusty bookcases in the chair's corner office at the MFA building, we noticed that the room had received some attention. It was freshly painted, but not too neatly, and overall, the rest of the departmental suite appeared dingy. A nondescript gray carpet had been repaired in places with duct tape. Although paint had been recently applied, in the walls of the chairman's office, here and there, a peculiar brown stain had seeped through. Although I later had thick industrial wallpaper applied, these dark stains inexorably appeared through the thick beige fabric from time to time. Given later events, this strange phenomenon put in mind *The Amityville Horror*.

This had been the office of the first two full-time surgical chairs at George Washington, Dr. Brian Blades and Dr. Paul Adkins. Both were fine men, but all of their predecessors prior to 1945 had been practitioners, not full-time academicians. Dr. Adkins, an inveterate cigarette smoker, as were many older thoracic surgeons, had died the year before from lung cancer, leaving vacant the chair to which I had been recruited. In spite of initial inauspicious appearances, I felt honored to occupy this office. I recalled vividly a statement of Dr. Blades, which had been a personal inspiration. Studying for surgical boards in the early morning hours, many years before in Cleveland, I came upon his words in his text on thoracic surgery, "It is a privilege to become a member of one of the greatest fraternities, the brotherhood of surgeons." His pronouncement bolstered my spirits considerably and I would recall these words when times were difficult. Yet, judging from letters remaining in the files, neither of my two predecessors had been happy or at all content. The old correspondence was depressing, particularly towards the end of their tenures. Peculiarly, files of former residents extended back only two or three years. Letters from the American Board of Surgery indicated that some had either not taken or had not passed Surgical Board examinations.

Opening the left-hand file drawer of the desk, I found several old copies of *Playboy,* a pack of Camel cigarettes, and an opened bottle of scotch whiskey. Somehow, these artifacts were comforting. My immediate predecessor had been at the least human. I had placed my leather folio on a corner table, and, looking up from the files, I noticed a roach crawling into its cleft. Shaking the creature to the floor, I now became concerned. My Nevada office was at least clean, though desert dust tended to accumulate. After touring the laboratories, John grumbled that little work was being done. I went to visit the dean's office in the hospital and John returned to the corner office to continue unpacking. When I returned, I found him sitting there, arms crossed, virtually on guard and scowling, "I don't know if this is such a good idea, Dr. DePalma, these people mean you no good." Apparently, while we were touring the facility, some office staff had tried to snoop through my files. I reassured John that this was a good move for us and urged him to take the car to look around for housing opportunities. The next morning, in Bethesda, Eve told me that during the night, she heard John crying in the guest bedroom. He did not want to take the laboratory job even though it paid more, telling me he would be "back in the ghetto again." Thus, I was forced to part company with my friend and collaborator. He returned to the University of Nevada as an EEO officer. In addition to losing John, another bad omen blemished the Washington move: my little Siamese chocolate point, Mali Ying, had died in Cleveland during minor surgery on her paws.

The surgical residency at George Washington had not only been placed on probation, it had been formally disapproved. I discovered this problem when one of my Nevada residents, a GWU Med School graduate, told me about it just six weeks before our move. Then, just days before we moved East, I learned of a visit to the Residency Review Committee in Chicago. An associate dean, trained as a cardiovascular surgeon, and the current acting surgical chair, a taciturn and phlegmatic general surgeon, assured me that the residency problem was easily correctable. This was a "paperwork matter" which they could easily sort out at the Chicago meeting. I had to ask to attend this meeting. The dean appeared nervous and defensive. I discovered that the residency problem was actually much more serious than I had been led to believe. Two well-respected surgical chairmen who had reviewed the program called me aside outside of the committee room to re-emphasize how serious the issues were. I was astonished. After all, this was the hospital that saved President Reagan. The residency would not be approved without restructuring. The problems were considered that grave. They were, as I later learned, exactly right.

We needed to begin recruiting residents within several months for the next academic year. I believed that the best way to deal with complicated challenges, no matter how onerous, is to generate enthusiasm for each part of the task. Gilbert Highet, professor of humanities at Columbia College, had said this and it stuck in my mind. Many boring tasks, he taught, must be done to clear hurdles toward greater things. A proposal for the Residency Review Committee requires the production of a document the size of a Metropolitan telephone book, much of it tedious boilerplate. But sandwiched between boilerplate, the program needed a substantive educational plan. The faculty at George Washington considered this exercise "paper work" of no real consequence and had not been able to produce a coherent document. Essentially, I needed to deal with this problem alone except for help from the residents themselves, and surprisingly, considerable support from the part-time faculty. Having just completed such an application two years before at the University of Nevada, I did not look forward to repeating this task, and had not been informed of this problem when I was recruited. Even more important than producing a document was making required programmatic changes. Such changes are painful and unpleasant for faculty and residents alike. Rather than being helpful during this process, the attitude of full-time faculty members was an impediment; they still believed that the residency was fine in its present state. This requirement was simply a matter of paper shuffling. I asked William Bishop, an educational consultant from Nevada, to help in formulating the proposal.

Impatience and righteous indignation are of no help in confronting problems, unless these can be used to motivate others. One of my own mentors had written of my own deficiencies in this regard, "He tolerates fools poorly." Initially, I took this as a compliment, but this trait is not an asset in a leader. What may seem foolish to some might simply be a different and even valid point of view. Clearly, there are also many fools who, somehow or other, need to be led. The existing surgical faculty, for the most part, lacked the academic motivations that drove me, and surgeons in the trenches of patient care can question these with some validity. Some were clearly respected practitioners, and unselfconscious about any lack of academic cachet. Full professors had written no more than eight or ten journal reports, most of these case descriptions. No coherent laboratory program existed in surgery, no one had earned a scientific grant of any consequence, nor was scholarly activity sincerely valued. Since the faculty had tenure and support in the dean's office, replacing them was not an option. Other candidates had been wise enough to figure this out before accepting this position, but I was beguiled by the prospect of a chairmanship in Washington, D.C., and also overconfident of my abilities to change these attitudes after the Nevada experience, where practicing surgeons valued research.

The shortcomings of that chairmanship could be easily understood in the light of past history. But I never reconciled my vision of a university department with that ingrained institutional culture, and as my ideals were challenged, I tried desperately to effect clearly impossible changes. This is a pitfall for any new leader. Such powerlessness, combined with a lack of local knowledge, can prove frustrating in the extreme. Incoming chairmen used to require and get the resignations of an entire faculty. They could then choose who was to stay. This process provided a mechanism for change (not always for the better) in many corporations as well as in the executive branches of government. Most of those who have to leave, successfully obtain other positions. This tradition had been lost in academic medicine. In any event, most faculty wanted to stay in Washington and had no option except private practice locally. And as much as they were unhappy with the institution, only one, during my tenure, exercised this option.

Residents and staff continually rehashed the treatment of President Ronald Reagan after he was shot at the Capital Hilton and rushed to the GW emergency room. That episode had been handled quite well. However, many claimed credits for its success, and, at the same time, as does happen in Washington, others apportioned retroactive blame. And subsequent statements and actions continued to tarnish that fine outcome. The thoracic surgeon who actually operated on Ronald Reagan, Dr. Benjamin Aaron, got little credit, and was later criticized for reasons that I could never fathom. Great credit was given to the surgeon inserting a chest tube in the emergency room, and there could be no doubt that he acted wisely in calling for prompt thoracic surgical intervention. The intervention itself recovered a "Devastator" bullet that had not detonated and the surgeon wisely removed the missile from the mediastinum. Later, the radiologist who interpreted X-rays showing a postoperative pneumonia celebrated himself along with the medical staff, making the momentous decision to start penicillin. The manner in which this case was discussed publicly appeared unseemly. The incident was well handled clinically, but pronounced needs for professional credit were uniquely part of the Washington scene. Anyone who operated upon, stood near, or even related to a prominent political figure, claimed glory. Physicians, including a thoracic surgeon who had nothing to do with the case, appeared on television to comment. Hyperbole is part and parcel of Potomac Fever. With the exception of the dean for clinical affairs, Dennis O'Leary, who early provided updates to a ravenous press during the acute episode, others came out of the woodwork seeking gratuitous attention. Similar television appearances, by people who had nothing to do with the incident, occurred as well when the President later had his colon removed at the Bethesda Naval Hospital.

Ultimately, this posturing destroyed the opportunity to benefit the medical center that worked hard to save our president. The George Washington University Hospital never received any notable funds or donations for this fine performance, in part, because of a negative comment in the *Los Angeles Times* about Reagan's policies by one of the surgical team when Reagan was running for re-election. The surgeon who attended him in the emergency room, a sincere and dedicated Democrat, believed that had Reagan's policies existed in the past, he would never have been able to attend medical school. The publicity that followed, irrespective of fact, was pure Washington partisan politics. After seeking and receiving permission from the doctor, administration publicists and the President stressed his ethnicity. After the doctor spoke to a liberal Hollywood personality, the story found its way into the *Los Angeles Times*. *The Washington Post* trumpeted the negative story with unfavorable references to Reagan's policies.

The dean for clinical affairs asked me, as an Italian American, to write an institutional letter of apology. Ronald Reagan's brief answer to my letter came by return mail, "Thank you for your kind letter. It was probably a bad idea. After all, we are all Americans." George Washington University Hospital did everything possible to obtain sorely needed donations in honor of the Reagans. The emergency room was named after him. The university president later invited the great communicator to discuss gun control and the Brady Bill, which he now supported. No substantial funds were donated to the needy George Washington University Hospital. But in the fall of 2000, I learned that a multimillion-dollar donation was made to the University of California in Reagan's name.

The Residency Review Committee document, which included necessary changes in resident staffing, was completed by November 1983. Not only was the surgical program inappropriately overstaffed, several residents had serious personal, professional or academic problems. With administrative support, we revised the program from five to six years to accommodate the extra residents as well as to provide a much needed research year. This would, in turn, attract better candidates. In retrospect, we might have been better off eliminating extra positions, ridding the program of marginal residents. This was more than a scheduling issue; some residents caused substantial clinical problems. Early in my experience, a resident assistant actually disrupted a splenorenal shunt in a critically ill patient after I left him to close the wound—one of the worst clinical experiences I had ever had. In another instance, I did not wish to recommend a resident for a clinical appointment in our Veterans Administration Hospital. This individual had a world-record number of written complaints, but the faculty went ahead with the recommendation without my approval. The resulting fracas almost cost me my position. A fine attorney, a liberal Democrat who had come to Washington with the Roosevelt New Deal, helped me survive.

The training program emerged from disapproval into probation. After re-examination at twelve months, we, then, were fully approved. With full approval, we attracted excellent young surgeons, including some former Nevada students. But the time spent in remedying the residency blunted my own research efforts. I was further crippled by not having John Wilburn to help me. The studies in experimental atherosclerosis, ended when the National Institutes of Health did not fund a new grant application with the radiology department. Ordinarily, I would have simply reapplied, but neither the time nor the encouragement was forthcoming. The vice president for medical affairs told me that placing a mechanical heart in Louisville, Kentucky was more of a surgical achievement than publishing scholarly articles in peer-reviewed journals. The heart implants proved to be short-lived.

A prominent Boston surgeon once stated that Washington, D.C., was, "Not exactly a center of surgical thought." Nor was it a center of technical brilliance. Operating times were, on average, longer than those in Cleveland and Nevada. However, in general, this was true along most of the East Coast. Residents were allowed to stumble through procedures and they regarded this as a right. Some operating room nurses were inattentive and undisciplined and some were unacceptably hostile. By and large, clinical outcomes were just what one might expect. A case presented at my first mortality conference was that of a thirty-seven-year-old woman who had died shortly after an operation for a perforated appendix. A resident had observed her for an extended period preoperatively. Having never seen a person of this age die of appendicitis, I was baffled and astonished. No one wanted to discuss the case openly. They claimed that they were under a "gag" order. The same resident soon presented me with a case of dead bowel, again after a prolonged period of observation. That patient died as well. I became even more cautious in my supervision of cases after these experiences, gun-shy really. The residents became annoyed with me because I did not "give them the case" as did other attending surgeons. Of course, I had been spoiled by the fine surgical teamwork we had in Cleveland and Nevada. If faced with adverse outcomes and systems problems, the best course is to request outside consultants. Out of a misguided sense of loyalty, I did not do this. I had been taught to tend to dirty laundry in-house.

The faculty-student ratio at the medical school was extreme. With 25 students rotating through short clerkship periods, it was difficult get to know each student, much less to exert an educational impact. The response to proposed change in student-faculty ratio was, "If we took ten less students, would your department like to take a three-hundred-thousand-dollar yearly cut?" George Washington and Georgetown both had the highest tuition costs in the United States. At that time, George Washington's tuition, about $30,000 per year, exceeded that of Georgetown. Most graduating students had accumulated large debts, therefore, finances played an important role in future career choices and, presumably, in subsequent billing behavior. Certainly, this institution, depending upon students' fees to support faculty salaries, tended toward a pre-Flexnerian model. Finance, not education or research, continued as an endless issue at almost all meetings. I had come East with reassurances that I might be able to establish a corporate departmental practice. This model could have helped both the practitioners and the institution but was patently impossible at that time. The suggestion had been naïve at best, and deceptive at worst.

Faculty income derived from three funding sources: medical school, hospital, and practice plan collection. The scheme looked good on paper, but the arrangement was that of "The Iron Pot." After being commingled centrally, funds were dispersed, after a charade of budget meetings to discuss allocations. Accounting was done on an accrual rather than on a cash basis. Individuals with barely a high school education handled collections. Neither my Nevada accountants nor I could comprehend the flow of funds, and I paid the Nevada accounting firm $500 for this honest opinion. Collections were notably poor, and overhead was notably high. After a busy first quarter with major vascular cases, I was surprised to get a skimpy bonus check equivalent to the amount collected for two major operations in Cleveland or in Nevada. I was earning less money than I had in Reno, certainly much less than what I had earned in Cleveland, and Washington was an expensive venue in many respects. Meanwhile, my former corporate practices in Cleveland and Nevada were prosperous and profitable.

Compared to national academic standards, surgical salaries were startlingly low. I could understand why the faculty groused continually, and I, as well as the institution, had disappointed them. The faculty hoped I might bring about a degree of financial independence but I never accomplished this. Cost reductions and certain efficiencies made things somewhat better. As a first step, I asked that the telephones be answered during business hours by a human being and that practitioners' telephones be cross-covered by secretaries rather than being placed on answering services. This met with considerable resistance from the secretarial staff. The year before I came, the department had spent more than it had earned. The accrual system then caught up and other departments had to make up surgery's loss by contributing to an already paid bonus pool. Mrs. Kathleen Lewis, our efficient departmental manager from Nevada, came to help with the support staff. Office personnel did not seem to work regular hours. A pregnant woman arrived at ten or eleven and went home at three in the afternoon doing little during this time. She had been hired as a surgical secretary and proved so inept that she was not allowed to answer the telephone. Kathleen carefully recorded her hours on a time card and we then paid her exactly for the time she had been present. She quit in a rage, accusing us of discrimination. We solved this problem by retroactively firing her so she could collect welfare. A senior secretary ultimately wanted to be let go under similar circumstances, so that she, too, would be eligible for welfare.

Strange events surfaced, and strange people came to see me in that corner office. A clinical professor, a plastic surgeon-lawyer who never operated, had been indicted for tax evasion and attempts to bribe federal officials. After serving his time in a federal facility, he petitioned to have his faculty appointment renewed. My negative decision was unpopular with his good friend, the "cardiovascular" dean. Other weird rumors and accusations included stories of piling up bills in desk drawers or collecting fees outside of the practice plan. A senior administrator asked me if I know how it was possible to cheat motion picture theaters by concealing ticket sales, something I had never really considered before. An oral surgeon was arrested for dissecting human fetuses in his garage. Some days, I dreaded to think what new and bizarre event would greet me at the stained corner office.

Within a day of my arrival, an effusive and seemingly well-intentioned faculty member appeared to tell me all about himself. A member of the prestigious University Surgeons, the only one other than I in the department, gave the appearance of a true believer in research and progress, and it was clear that he truly believed much of what he told me. With a gleam in his eyes, he told me that University Surgeons was planning a meeting at our institution the next year, which he had personally arranged. With more enthusiasm than prudence, I called the president of our learned society, who groaned when I mentioned this person. The society was meeting elsewhere that next year, and I should have known that these meetings were arranged three years in advance. I felt foolish and chastened. Dealing with this individual was like taking a trip down the rabbit hole with Alice—"curioser and curioser." Somehow, he convinced himself of the truth behind his statements, of which most were pure fantasies. Oddly, in spite of his criticism to me that the rest of the faculty was non-academic, such was his charm and radiant goodwill that faculty, the residents, and particularly the "cardiovascular" dean supported him. They had written several papers together. I was alternately complimented or chided on my "handling" of him.

He flitted about, Peter Pan-like, to national and international surgical meetings, and I got negative comments about his claims and academic presentations. Some nationally prominent people told me that something was wrong. I tended to shrug these criticisms off as a species of activity not uncommon in academic surgery. Some individuals were actually making a living of sorts on the lecture circuit. More seriously, however, I was also told of his many negative statements about my leadership style. Generally, I do not wish to intrude upon colleagues, believing that with time and patience, many settle down as they have much to lose. But this is not always the case and did not happen in this instance. Most serious were allegations of billing for cases that he did not attend in the operating room. Eventually, the chief of staff of the hospital forced the credentials committee to reappraise his application for transplant surgical privileges, which I would not approve. The executive committee ended his surgical activities, which had already cost our self-insured malpractice fund three million dollars. His supporters then accused me of carrying on a "vendetta," a charge rapidly countered by my asking if this was an ethnic slur. One of my rules of chairmanship became: "The first person to come to your office will probably cause the most trouble." Another rule, particularly true in Washington, is: "For every action, there is an equal and opposite reaction." Oddly enough, this individual, along with the world-record complaint residents, tried to accuse me of unnecessary surgery when I advised an early operation on a possible appendicitis which was done by a new junior faculty member. In spite of this, I had had hopes of redemption for him, but was told by the credentials committee that redemption was really a matter for the next world.

After those first years, and with the exodus of marginal residents, things appeared to improve. With the residency program fully approved, residents were now publishing creditable research. We had a large number of qualified applicants and hospital occupancy was high. Our kidney transplant service, directed by Dr. Said Karmi and Dr. Anne Thompson, chief of nephrology, was thriving. I had requested and had received serious consideration for a helicopter service to bring outlying trauma and critically ill patients to our hospital. After much discussion, this could be not accomplished. Administration was certain that we had enough patients to fill the beds, but this condition did not last long. Our Foggy Bottom neighbors did not want helicopters landing in the hospital parking lot; most important were difficulties in routing helicopters in the White House flight zone. The trauma service increasingly became a matter of treating inner city "Rod and Gun Club" members. One of the team members that saved President Reagan recused himself from the trauma service to pursue his own interests. I remained among five general surgeons rotating on this service. I kept a small apartment, a pied a terre, close by on Pennsylvania Avenue. On call nights, I could relax, knowing that I could get to the hospital quickly, as I did in Cleveland and Nevada. On several occasions involving hemorrhage control, this helped.

Negativism permeated the institution. The dean that had hired me left under fire. I was vocal about how good things had been out West. No one really cares how things were at your last position. This type of grousing is always an error. Just after my arrival in Washington, an administrative dean told me that the search process for my position had not been properly carried out. Compared to the West, I had expected that Washington would be an administrative paradise. Its pervasive inefficiency in many areas amazed and irritated me. I offered to return to Nevada in the white Mercedes, and this would have been a wise move. I heard no more about the search problems. At the same time, Dr. John Cameron left Baltimore for the chair at Vanderbilt in Nashville. He encountered insoluble problems and simply returned to Johns Hopkins. His step required the dimension of insight, moral courage, and support that I lacked. I felt that the alternative in insoluble situations is to do what Harry Truman did with his World War I goof-up-artillery company. He graciously accepted the shortcomings existing among his troops and succeeded brilliantly. I tried that and failed.

Negativity and cynicism are fatal in individuals as well as in institutions. Great institutions may be considered as the lengthening shadows of great men, and, an association with great institutions tends to create great individuals. But at George Washington Medical School, at that time, the organizational structure and widespread cynicism caused failure of what should have been, and in some ways was an outstanding medical center. Pettiness, backbiting, second-guessing and lack of collegial support, and envy tended to dominate conversations. The medical service did not respect the surgical service. There existed, as in other university systems, but to a greater degree, poorly disguised disdain for surgeons. This attitude, in my opinion, dooms any center aspiring to world-class status. Surgeons capable of delivering the best outcomes have founded virtually all of our great clinics. Achieving outstanding surgical results requires intelligence and discipline. Medically oriented administrators sometimes fail to recognize this. At one time or another, most of us will need some kind of surgical procedure. Favorable outcomes depend upon good judgment, timely referral and expeditious, well-done technical procedures. When financial motives drive institutional policy and practice, surgeons need to review indications and results carefully and objectively. On the other hand, failed surgeons may not be the best candidates for leadership.

Orthopedics had become a separate department for reasons I never understood, and further, did not want a plastic surgeon in our department to have privileges to perform hand surgery. I returned urgently from an overseas meeting to mediate a mean-spirited public dispute acted out in a meeting of the entire medical staff. The ugly episode ended when the young plastic surgeon threatened to sue the orthopedists. He was criticized severely for that, and later left to enter private practice. Disenchantment and cynicism marred the correspondence and speech of senior clinicians, though many were outstanding individuals. A paucity of peer reviewed research grants plagued the basic science departments, and clinicians resented contributing practice income to support the basic science faculty teaching the two preclinical years. Some clinicians suggested that the clinical faculty might just as well teach the basic sciences.

Governance was essentially monolithic. The vice president for medical affairs was the chief operating officer responsible for all elements of the center: the hospital, the medical school, faculty practice plan, and faculty medical associates. Three associate deans, one for clinical affairs, essentially the chief of staff of the hospital, one academic dean for the medical school, and one dean for administration, completed his staff. This structure, with its original complement, worked, after a fashion, but one could sense the potential problems with this stovepipe structure when the CEO was weak or had bad judgment. When I first arrived, Dennis O'Leary, the dean for clinical affairs, was of great help. The administrative dean, Philip Birnbaum, accurately predicted a failing financial future, and recommended early the sale of the hospital. The "cardiovascular" dean, confined to the medical school, was innocuous though not popular with students who felt him deceptive. Given his perceptions about the problems of the surgical residency, the students were exactly right. When he succeeded as vice president for medical affairs, I resolved to support him, though several clinical chairs objected to this appointment.

The leadership decided assignment for all Medicare cases, and initially, the cardiac surgeon and I opposed this. We believed that individuals ought to have the responsibility for paying their own bills, clearly an impractical view since downtown Washington patients often kept their Medicare checks. However, my initial objection, short term, was incorrect. Accepting Medicare assignment sharply boosted collections, but with time, Medicare reimbursements were drastically reduced. Administration then insisted upon raising clinical fees to support its failing hospital. By law, we were now obliged to collect the 20% deduction from poor Medicare patients. As the hospital gradually became an inner city institution, more practice income had to be diverted into its support. The municipal hospital, DC General Hospital, first closed itself to trauma cases and finally closed completely. George Washington University Hospital lost ten to thirty million dollars in each of two years, while bed occupancy declined. Similar things were happening in other urban university hospitals, including Georgetown, which progressed downward, at a parallel but slower rate. Paradoxically, hospitals in the DC Metropolitan area that did not interfere or tax physician income, such as Sibley and The Washington Hospital Center, continued to thrive.

Surgery at George Washington had built a successful kidney transplantation program, and with the prospect of Medicare support, I was convinced that we could develop equally successful liver and pancreas transplant programs. Shortly, consultants, most of them younger than our residents, wearing Rolex watches and costly Tiffany gold, visited the department. The new vice president called them to look into the financial feasibility of an expanded transplant program. I learned from the consultants that the hospital had failed to collect the Medicare fees for kidney transplants for several years. The consultants innocently asked me what we, the practice group, could do about this. Our department had collected professional fees, but due to sheer neglect, the hospital administration had not collected payments due.

In Cleveland, when we were engaged in serious yacht-racing competition, we privately named one crew member "the port-starboard man." This was a person, who, when asked which tack to take, was always exactly wrong, but we always treated him kindly. If we did the opposite of what he recommended, we were almost always right. George Washington had precisely the same problem with its VP for medical affairs, except that he was now captain of the ship. After grooming outstanding young surgeons for liver transplants, the port-starboard vice president decided that we should not expand our transplantation program. Both young surgeons soon left.

Other potential good moves were thwarted. One of these was approval by the residency review committee for our residents to work at nearby Sibley Hospital This was a much better option than our existing affiliation with a private hospital outside the beltway, which would not grant the GW faculty admitting privileges. I also came to believe that our residents were learning some bad habits and shortcuts at that affiliated hospital. George Washington, with its complement of highly capable house staff, clearly had the capability to handle complicated problems. Simple hernias and gallbladders could be done in any community hospital. The Sibley affiliation was vetoed, as the "Port-Starboard Man" believed that income would be lost. However, "bread and butter" surgery continued being done in increasing numbers in community hospitals. Another promising plan was to develop to a clinic-type arrangement. We visited the Ochsner Clinic in New Orleans, the Lamb Clinic in Albuquerque and the Cottage Hospital Group in Santa Barbara. This was a fine idea, but once again, negativism prevailed, citing difficulty in attracting paying patients to downtown Washington, even with the special expertise we could offer. This obstacle could have been overcome as other inner city clinics had accomplished this using well-organized security measures. But when wife of one of my patients was mugged outside the intensive care unit, important referral sources from Virginia vanished, and I became discouraged. Administration ignored complaints of roaches in the rooms and bad staff attitudes. After several patients complained about roach infestation, one of my favorite floor nurses from Alabama would reassure me, "Now, don't y'all worry, Raaff. I got roach motels in them rooms." Other major institutions such as Johns Hopkins and the Cleveland Clinic managed to overcome similar inner-city problems, but George Washington University Hospital at that time did not appear able to accomplish this task.

When DC General limited admissions, trauma victims and drug addicts deluged the emergency room. The infectious disease group became quite expert in treating HIV infections, but some staff viewed the presence of AIDS patients as a liability. Misguided attitudes of political correctness and a scarcity of private rooms prevented meaningful progress in dealing effectively with the needs of these unfortunate patients. I acquired a substantial experience in operations on HIV-positive patients, with good results. The patients were quite grateful. Small advances continued to give me hope. When I first arrived, the operating rooms were dirty. Little scraps of hair, suture and detritus lurked in corners of the operating suites. I had never seen anything like this before; neither had a newly recruited head operating room nurse, an Asian American Mormon lady from Salt Lake City. She insisted having the rooms cleaned up. In the course of accomplishing changes, she encountered fierce opposition, and, ultimately, in establishing discipline, she terminated some nurses. When she left, the operating room environment reverted to its former state.

There are good things about a position in Washington, D.C., and after a while, I understood why many who came here wanted to stay. The city itself was architecturally and intellectually inspiring. One had the sense, perhaps inflated, of doing important things in an important place. I attended services at the National Cathedral, praying that we could ultimately draw upon the spirit of the great cathedral to help establish a first-rate medical institution in the nation's capital. A nucleus of talented African Americans work in the district. Many of them cheerfully made everything work, including operating rooms, my clinic, as well as receptions on Capitol Hill. One dark and stormy Halloween night, I was called to the White House to suture a minor injury on an important person who did not wish to come to the clinic. As I walked out the door, my chief clinic nurse shoved a paper bag in my hand. It contained fine nylon suture materials. I told her that the White House dispensary was supposed to have everything that I needed. She laughed, "Doc DePalma, just take the bag." She was perfectly right; the White House dispensary had coarse silk suture material and no Mayo stand.

The practice in erectile dysfunction grew extensively. The

institutional resources helped screen over 1,700 men through its vascular laboratory and radiology department. Urology, endocrinology, and neurology enhanced this effort, along with a talented microvascular surgeon, Dr. Michael Olding. Our group defined the efficacy of surgery for large and small vessel disease causing impotence. While only about 7% of men became surgical candidates, we learned that most of these men could be treated medically. A comment was made that the amount of surgery we attracted was disappointing. More than the usual complement of nervous men could be found in the Washington environment, but most often, erectile dysfunction had a physical basis. In 1994, we published a definitive report outlining this experience. Our expertise in vascular disease and the treatment of erectile dysfunction generated invitations to share our experience at home and abroad, including China, India, England, France, Czechoslovakia, Italy, Greece, and Brazil. Sadly, I was out of the country in India when my good friend, John Wilburn, died in Cleveland after cardiac surgery.

The Cosmos club was another bright aspect of the Washington scene. The club had in its membership bright and interesting people from diverse disciplines. I came to respect the intellectual integrity and the high standards of fellow club members while serving on its admissions committee. I remained a member while living in Nevada, and my two daughters had elegant wedding receptions at the club. The Washington Academy of Surgery with Drs. LaSalle Leffall, chief of surgery at Howard University and Robert Wallace, chief at Georgetown generously collaborated in citywide resident research presentations at the club. This meant a great deal to these young investigators as altruism and intellectual integrity characterized the atmosphere there.

Altruism and a keen sense of justice also characterized a young district prosecutor. An earnest young woman appeared in my office one afternoon to ask me to testify in the case of a gunshot wound. The victim, a drug dealer, had been shot with an Uzi automatic weapon, and, at four in the morning, I had helped the residents remove his spleen and clean up wounds near his femoral artery.

The orthopedic team had also debrided a wound on his knee. He had several varieties of retained bullets, including .38 and .45 caliber and 9mm bullets along with old and new entry and exit wounds. The surgical residents, expert in penetrating trauma, easily identified each missile. The police had caught the shooters and the prosecutor needed me to testify that his current injury, as opposed to the others, could have been fatal. Although the wound of the spleen was obviously potentially fatal, because of the previously retained fragments, she said, the case required a personal court appearance. The demand seemed excessive, but I agreed to appear. My senior resident at that time, also a highly motivated young woman, constructed a cardboard mannequin showing locations and entry sites of all wounds including the ones we had treated. The two of them coached me to memorize each of the sites and its associated missiles. Of course, the whole thing was silly, but then Washington is, above all, a city of lawyers and I felt that she was quite sincere in seeing that justice was done

Postoperatively, I had found the patient holding court with two good-looking, honey-skinned women hovering about him. Dressed in silk pajamas and an Italian designer's bathrobe, he expansively flashed a great roll of bills. The hospital would never collect a cent for his care nor would our staff be paid for staying up all night with him. I told him about the seriousness of his injuries, and he assured me, "Doc, it is just a matter of business." I said, "Well, I think you had better change the corner on which you do business." When I told him that we were going to court because they had arrested his attackers, he shrugged indifferently.

The young prosecutor arrived at our Pennsylvania Avenue office building exactly on time, on the court date, with a car and driver. Sitting dejectedly in the backseat, she told me that my patient had been shot again, this time, fatally. Nevertheless, she still wanted me to testify. I waited in a room along with three tough DC detectives in pork pie hats, who told me that juveniles had been assigned as shooters because they would not receive a death penalty or a severe sentence. They complained about the absence of a death penalty in the District of Columbia. On the stand, following the young lawyer's lead, I solemnly described each past and present gunshot wound along with their potential complications. The defendants were four adolescent African Americans, ranging from thirteen to sixteen years of age. They giggled and pointed as we enumerated each injury and each type of bullet. Apparently, these youngsters had done all of the shooting, and each was pointing to his particular hits. The orthopedic surgeon had refused to testify, and I regretted my participation in this sad exercise. I later suggested that we discontinue, or at least minimize, our trauma service to concentrate on elective surgery—recommendations that were neither politically correct nor well received.

I resigned as chairman of surgery in the midst of a faculty exodus in the spring of 1992. The chairman of anesthesia, a close personal friend, resigned first. The chairman of neurosurgery, whom we had gone to great pains to recruit, also resigned. Prior to my resignation, while I was in Puerto Rico giving an invited lecture series, the VP for medical affairs had announced his own resignation. I called to ask if there was anything I could do to help and his response was angry and distant. On my return, the VP told me that, in his opinion, I really had not done a good job and that the institution would be best served by my departure. I could have easily ignored his impulsive demand, as he himself was leaving. He had gone through this exact dialogue with another chairman who refused to resign. But I immediately wrote a letter of resignation. Perhaps, I should have stopped to consider this action, but this conversation with the "Port-Starboard Man" was an outrage. He was trying to blame others for his own failures. In that instant I perceived that, given the institutional history and damage already done, there was little further that I could contribute. However, for some time, I continued to reconsider how I might have done better to help this historic medical institution succeed. There are lessons to be learned in failures. My friends have reassured me that not much more could have been done. I am unaccustomed to failure and continued to view the institutional failure as a personal one. A surgical chairman was then appointed, without a national search, from within the existing faculty. The telephones in the department immediately returned to answering services.

Many university medical centers now teeter on the slippery slope of failure. Severe financial problems plaguing the current health care environment overshadow traditional university research and educational obligations. The idea that practice income and tuition can support a medical school is a serious error. This is not a good time for a medical school to own or try to run a hospital. Pragmatism suggests that one person can do little to reverse global trends, but certain individuals profoundly influence organizational outcomes. Notable successes do exist on the academic scene. Those personally failing in organizational situations are given to blaming others and external factors rather than themselves, and my own iteration of these events gives me pause. I was unusually optimistic about George Washington and tried to maintain that optimism right up to that final conversation with the "Port-Starboard Man." While I regard my efforts of that decade a failure, the faculty was kind enough to name an annual research lectureship after me. As can be seen from this account, the very ideals that guided me also failed to protect me.

The university president urged me to stay on, explaining that the hospital was "a conundrum" which needed to be relocated to Virginia. At the same time, President Trachtenberg, a Columbia College graduate, greatly improved the undergraduate program of the university. Its law school remains outstanding, but that professional faculty never suffered with a "practice plan" similar to that of the medical school. Lawyers tend to do well in Washington. After I left, George Washington Hospital was sold to a private corporation, which, on a hopeful note, built a new facility. I found the emergency room care to be excellent just recently. Medical students now rotate more at other sites and the Medical Faculty Association has separated from university control. A transplant program no longer exists, but the residency program remains approved. The research year for residents continues to be supported, but research residents are now filling in for shortened resident hours demanded by new regulations. Looking back, the attempt to meld individual ideals, no matter how high-minded, with institutional dynamics, can be dangerous. However damaging a struggle to fulfill these ideals, and however bloodied one may become in the process, the attempt is worth the pain. Change for the better only comes from groups of like-minded people working in concert, and these individuals comprise institutions. Sometimes, such ideas change the world. Sometimes they do not. Whatever the outcome, it is better to have tried and failed than to settle for passivity and inaction.

RIYADH TO RENO

The opposite of a profound truth
may well be another profound truth.
Niels Bohr

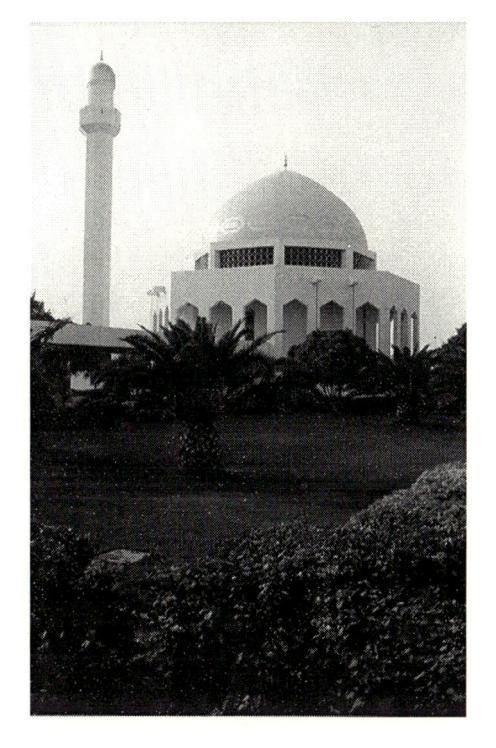

Mosque at the King Fahad Hospital in Saudi Arabia

After the chairmanship at George Washington, I spent several months, in 1993, directing surgery at the Fahad Hospital in Riyadh, Saudi Arabia. Saudi patients in Washington had recommended that I look into this post and I was interested in seeing, firsthand, another culture with viewpoints so different from ours. I was also becoming bored with what essentially was private practice at George Washington University. After a physical examination and an obligatory HIV test, I was given a visa to travel.

I learned that one does not travel to the Kingdom as a tourist. In the early summer of 1993, I left the heat and humidity of the District of Columbia for the dry blazing heat of Riyadh. Once the decision was made, they wanted me to travel within hours, rather than waiting a day or two to travel directly on a Saudi Air flight. I was booked on Lufthansa via Frankfurt. They apparently wanted me urgently. The Lufthansa flight went from Dulles to Frankfurt, and then, after a long layover, on to the Riyadh airport, a remarkable structure designed as a series of tents. I had traveled for over twenty-six hours and upon leaving the terminal at four in the morning, a furnace like a blast of dry heat struck me almost like a blow. A Sudanese driver took me to quarters at the hospital compound. By ten in the morning, the temperature was 120 degrees Fahrenheit with a relative humidity of about 10%. The architecture was designed to protect inhabitants from the sun: windows were slit-like, and buildings with crenelated walls appeared surreal. Some places looked like scenes of a *Star Wars* set. Men at the airport, save for the military, wore robe-like traditional garb, the *thobe*, and headgear which not only shielded the face but prevented evaporation of fluid into the dry air. I learned that men dressed similarly to be equal in the eyes of Allah. Distinctive or gold jewelry was not worn, though some men displayed an expensive fountain pen. The only thing that might distinguish a royal was a thin silver thread in the headgear. I had a platinum Rolex watch with the Saudi emblem, a gift from a patient. Men did not wear gold watches.

The National Guard Hospital, in the outskirts of the city, had volunteered and paid to be inspected by the American Joint Commission on Hospital Accreditation. They had received a certificate attesting to their status. The Joint Commission then reconsidered their policy of inspection of foreign hospitals, deciding that they were not empowered to grant overseas certification. The hospital had already framed its certificate in gold, proudly displaying it in its white-marble lobby. Hospital administration refused to return its trophy. The Fahad Hospital, an extensive complex, encircled a well-tended central garden with a fountain.

There were separate dining facilities for men and women; the sexes were segregated at meal times. The single-story building complex spread out extensively and was, in every respect, clean—almost sparkling—and quite modern. The hospital was staffed by a multinational group of surgeons: Swedish, Finnish, Egyptian, Pakistani, and Canadian. The resident staff, mainly Saudis, included a young woman. The residents accepted guidance, worked conscientiously, and many of them came to ask about obtaining further training in the United States. Seeing that they arrived quite late in the morning, I mentioned that if they wanted an American residency, they would have to be up by at least six in the morning. Morning rounds were to be completed before going to the operating room. Their eyes widened as I explained this, and most complied, though the lady resident, who was driven to the hospital in a Cadillac usually got in at about nine in the morning. Decades later, when GW had some Saudi residents, one of them told me that I had been a "legend" with this "inhuman" demand. But he and a few others did get residency positions in Washington, D.C. As a group, they said little and rarely questioned authority; they followed orders unquestioningly, possibly with an excess of zeal. Some seemed to flatter to the point of obsequiousness.

Saudi administrators conducted budget meetings dressed in traditional Arab garb, but the chief of staff told me that he did not approve of doctors dressing in thobe as the garment might inhibit emergency responses. Budget requests were considered carefully and funds, which appeared abundant, seemed to be wisely spent. Many administrators had MBAs earned in the United States, and budget-meeting deliberations were mercifully brief. These people did not bicker over minor issues as I had experienced in previous hospital committees in Washington. Once they made a decision, prompt and even impulsive action followed. Certain decisions were postponed with the words *"Bukara, In'sh'Allah*, tomorrow, perhaps or God willing." Individual Saudis offered thoughtful and generous hospitality. Well-trained English nursing sisters and a fine anesthesia staff completed the professional milieu. However, outside the hospital Compound, the environment was alien and threatening in a curious way. After my arrival, the personnel officer asked me to turn over my passport for some sort of Saudi ID. I refused to do this, kept my passport, and heard nothing more about the matter. They were kind enough to give me a car with some Arabic characters, which got me through checkpoints with a salute.

In one way, I felt that I was not giving them the kind of service that I should have as the kind of vascular cases that I usually cared for were rare. Carotid atherosclerosis, aneurysms, or patients with aortoiliac disease were not in evidence. At the King Faisal Hospital in downtown Riyadh, I saw inflammatory arteritides in consultation with a staff vascular surgeon who had been trained in Canada. He told me that he did see enough atherosclerosis among the city dwellers to keep him busy. The population of city dwellers in central Riyadh differed compared to the Fahad on the edge of town, serving the National Guard. Atherosclerotic disease was rare and smoking was uncommon. In contrast, diabetes was common, and patients demonstrated a unique peripheral pattern of calcification involving the vessels of the hands, feet and even the penis. In contrast to my experience in the United States, most of these individuals successfully healed distal toe or midfoot amputations. These amputations were often done without recourse to arteriography. To humor me, the staff obtained some arteriograms showing perfectly clean distal vessels in the lower extremities. Trauma, renal failure and a high prevalence of cirrhosis related to hepatitis were important surgical challenges. My operative work consisted mainly of routine general surgery, laparoscopic cholecystectomy and kidney transplants for a large pool of patients on dialysis. Transplant procedures were often done on several patients as kidneys became available immediately following automobile or truck accidents. Just after I left Fahad in the fall of 1993, a team led by a Saudi surgeon, trained by Startzl in Pittsburgh, performed the first liver transplant in the Kingdom. I had encouraged him to keep working in the laboratory to develop the team's skills rather than taking routine surgical calls. Interestingly, this young surgeon, who wore traditional garb, also mentioned that his fellowship at Pittsburgh had been "almost inhuman." I had long wanted George Washington

University to accomplish hepatic transplantation, but this did not and still has not happened. The Fahad team's achievement reflected considerable technical skill and expertise carried out by clever, determined people.

After several months, when I was planning a trip home, an earnest young physician entreated me to stay on as permanent chief. While I enjoyed the clinical environment, had a fine place to live, and a butler who took good care of me, I was ambivalent about remaining in the Kingdom. I waffled, repeating to him, "In'sh'Allah, God willing," words Saudis themselves used meaning, "Perhaps." As I uttered this phrase, the man's face darkened. He said that I had truly invoked God's will. If I were lying, I would be punished. "Allah knew what was in our hearts." His words were spoken bitterly and his concern and anger were real; I was in conversation with a zealot and I, an infidel, had given offense. I had encountered Islam and I reflected that the dates on our X-ray films read 1414. Possibly, I had now acquired a potentially ferocious enemy. I tried to reassure him that I was really thinking over a return. I recalled the words of the leader of the founding clan, Abdul Aziz. In wars uniting the Kingdom in the early 1900s, he recalled a victory over a member of a rival clan: "I struck him first on the leg and disabled him, quickly after that I struck at the neck; the head fell to one side and blood spurted up like a fountain: the third blow at the heart, I saw the heart, which was cut in two, palpitate . . . It was a joyous moment. I kissed the sword." (From Robert Lacey, *The Kingdom: Arabia and the House of Sa'ud*.)

Early morning prayer and the lilting chants from the minarets four times called everyone to pray, "Allah Akbar, Allah is Great." The reminders were impressive and almost hypnotic, but prayer times were not observed universally within the hospital. Outside of the hospital environment, everything and everyone stopped during prayer. Merchant owners left their precious gold and fine precious stones untended, or perhaps covered with a velvet cloth, while they went to the mosque. No one stole from them; the penalty was amputation of the right hand at the wrist. For adultery the penalty remained death and beheadings for serious crimes occurred once a week in the center square of Riyadh. Although I was regularly prodded to attend, as were other Westerners, I avoided those events. Social interactions could be awkward and, at times, discomforting. At a dinner, the American wife of an Islamic host chided me for offering to shake her hand. She touched no man but her husband. At some dinners, the company was that of men. Wives were never seen nor introduced. The Gulf War had just ended and hulks of Scud missiles were still about. Curiously, some men expressed admiration for Saddam Hussein and the secular society surviving in Iraq, while others looked forward to visiting their "cousins," their former allies in Israel. Such contradictory attitudes were openly shared in these gatherings. The lack of alcoholic beverages bothered me little at all, but some Westerners brewed vile homemade beverages using stills openly sold in the local supermarket. The women shopping there wore *abayas*, or head coverings, and always had their husbands with them. Women were not allowed to drive cars nor were unmarried couples allowed to travel or publicly dine together. Some of the Western wives with children frankly enjoyed the culture and were pleased about the absence of drugs and crime. Many staff wives spent the summer away in Crete or Malta, and there were some, including my wife, who did not wish to come at all.

Magazines showed crudely censored photographs, an arm here, a leg there, and parts of the female torso. For a Christian, even a relaxed one such as I, the strictures on religious expression were troublesome. Crosses, religious services and certain classical recordings were forbidden. Signs scrawled on desert rocks read: "Death to Christians." These messages, as opposed to casual graffiti in Western cities, appeared deadly serious. I had avoided religious discussions, as the chair of medicine at George Washington had counseled wisely that we went there as "mercenaries, not missionaries." However, while mediating a minor administrative dispute, I mentioned that I was a Christian and recommended "turning the other cheek." I was admonished that, in Islam, this is a sign of weakness. The ferocity and the implied violence of this judgment were disturbing. When I had decided to return home, a surgeon and his girlfriend attended a farewell dinner in the hospital compound. They offered to drive me to the airport, but then word came from hospital administration. We were told that I should not travel with this unmarried couple as the police might be looking to arrest us. My colleague drove me to the terminal alone. Just before he left, the Canadian chief of hospital security had hired a taxi to drive him around Riyad while he took unauthorized photographs. He was reported and detained for this offense.

In early fall, a call came from Reno to Riyadh, and it became evident that the nature of our telephone conversation was known. Calls coming through the hospital switchboard were monitored. I learned that the Veterans Administration Hospital had temporarily discontinued major thoracic and vascular surgery, jeopardizing the University of Nevada's residency program. Miles Standish, the genial associate dean and an old friend, suggested I consider a position in Reno. On my return to the United States, I met with the director of the VA hospital, Mr. Gary Whitfield, Dean Robert Daugherty, and Dr. Alex Little, the surgical chairman in Las Vegas who had salvaged our residency program. Dr. Little brought with him an important academic influence to Las Vegas from the University of Chicago. They offered appointments as chief of surgery at the Reno VA Hospital, vice chairman of surgery and associate dean at the medical school. I accepted their generous offer, but had to delay my departure from Washington for a week to cover the patient of a colleague who became ill during an aneurysm repair.

I was delighted to return to Nevada with its assurance of personal freedom as well as the open, tolerant atmosphere of our American West. But this, also, was a place of direct and simple justice, where the attorney general, a liberal Democrat, might carry a pistol in her purse and be present in Carson City to ensure an execution of a righteous death penalty. In 1997, an offer came to revisit Saudi Arabia to consider the chair at the King Faisal Hospital. The financial incentives offered were considerable. I found myself thinking about the Kingdom once again, and although housing was offered in the Diplomatic Compound, a privileged site, I realized that I did not wish to revisit Riyadh. The Silver State, in a sense, the antithesis of Saudi Arabia, was to be my home for several more years. Yet, the two places had similarities. Although Nevada was the first state to grant women the right to vote, it was, in its own way, a man's place. There were also women who did not wish to live there. Both places had desert environments, but the deserts of the Arabian Peninsula were absolutely stark and threatening, while the snow-capped peaks of Northern Nevada provided refreshing visual and temperate relief and Las Vegas shone like a jewel in the Southern Desert. I would not miss the undercurrents of intrigue and gossip in Washington or the controversies of the Middle East, nor did I miss tabouli or hummus.

Before leaving the District of Columbia, I contacted friends in vascular surgery at Northwestern, Iowa, and Colorado. I drove west on Route 80 across the country, this time in an Infiniti Q45, which replaced the dull diesel Mercedes that took me east in 1982. I stopped at the Cleveland Clinic where a Lebanese colleague had his third coronary revascularization. He was a much-loved gentleman and Prince Bandar flew up in a U.S. Air Force jet to visit. I sat with his family and friends as he recovered. Then, I visited Northwestern in Chicago, enjoying the forthright hospitality of Dr. Jimmy Yao and his wife, Louise. It was a short drive to the University of Iowa to see Dr. John Corson, chief of vascular surgery there. Driving further west, I dropped south off Route 80 into Denver to visit an old friend from Spain, Mrs. Reine Brickell, and spend a day with the thoughtful Dr. Robert Rutherford at the University of Colorado. During this cross-country trip, I recalled Dr. Brian Blades' words about the company of surgeons. It was a privilege to be among them.

After a night in Grand Junction and a spectacular drive through the Monument Desert, the Infiniti glided into shining Salt Lake City. The journey the next day from Salt Lake to Reno took only twelve hours, the Q45 clocking 140 miles an hour at 4500 rpm on straight stretches. The speedometer redlined at 6500. When I purchased this car, the dealer in Virginia offered to add a spoiler on the trunk. I now wished that I had accepted his offer. A spoiler on a sedan might be viewed as an affectation, but the dealer had been quite right. At the high speeds easily achieved by this vehicle, the rear end floated off the road. The Q car was no ordinary sedan. Nevada used to have no speed limit in the desert, but now, the state does. Approaching some road construction, a lone state trooper waved at me to slow down. He was grinning, and I think he understood how much fun it was to handle that fine machine on a straight well-paved road in the great desert. I stopped for lunch at Millie's Diner in Battle Mountain and could barely finish a generous juicy hamburger.

I passed the Mustang Ranch, an equivalent Western seraglio, shortly arriving in Reno at dusk. I turned off Route 80 and climbed southwest on McCarran Boulevard with the Mount Rose, still snow-capped, in view. It was a cool high desert evening, and I was elated to be back breathing fresh mountain air. I drove up to my house in the foothills at 2001 Lakeridge Drive, a place that Kathleen Lewis, in her inimitably efficient fashion, had found for me. Once again, I was home in the Silver State. I slept soundly and without moving until dawn.

A LIFE OF THE MIND

> The great doctor, Aquapendente being a famed surgeon and anatomist, should content himself . . . among his scalpels and ointments without trying to effect cures by medicine, as if a knowledge of surgery destroyed and opposed . . . a knowledge of medicine.
> Galileo

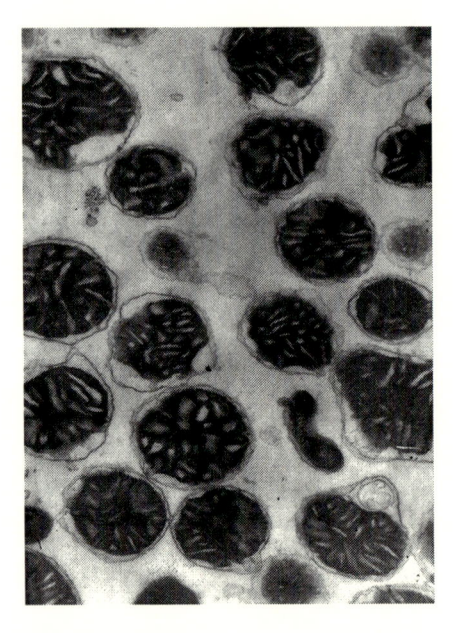

Electron Micrograph of isolated mitochondria

I once imagined that scholars worked in picturesque settings protected from worldly concerns. Universities long past were ecclesiastic institutions that focused upon scholarly inquiry. Maranon, the great Spanish internist and scholar, said that corporations lasted for decades, nations were meant for the centuries, but universities were created for the millennia. He was then dean of the University of Salamanca, an institution founded in A.D. 600, which spanned Moorish and Christian eras in Spain.

Ancient universities preserved the world's store of knowledge during the Dark Ages and Salamanca had passed on its heritage of Arabic advances in algebra, astronomy and medicine. The idea of working in a scholarly community, contemplating millennial concepts, appeared quite attractive to me. But modern university environments, I discovered, deviate from this ideal. The world is now deeply entrenched within the groves of academe. While scholarly instincts persist in a frenetic modern environment, the goals of scholars in academic medicine have become chaotic and confusing. These doctors attempt basic research along with a high level of competent practice, and surgeons, in particular, face an even more difficult challenge.

Surgical research does more than discover novel surgical techniques or devices. It also delves into diverse aspects of physiology, cell biology, biochemistry, and, lately, genetics. The idea of surgical scholarship, on the surface, might appear contradictory. A surgeon is considered to be a worker with his hands, and needs to balance scholarship with practice demands that take him away from books, and laboratory benches and into operating theaters. Some consider surgeons as procedure-oriented technicians. Scientific papers in surgical journals may be less widely acclaimed in scientific circles, while more Ph.D.'s now serve on research committees and write grant proposals essential to fund research enterprises. Surgeons contributed significantly to the medical progress of the twentieth century and continue to contribute at the beginning of the twenty-first century. Nobel Prizes have been awarded to surgeons,—to Alexis Carrel for vascular anastomoses, to Joseph E. Murray for transplantation, and to Charles B. Huggins for showing the hormonal effect upon prostate cancer. In addition to breathtaking advances in surgical technique, for example cardiopulmonary bypass and cardiac surgery, surgeons achieved spectacular advances in nutrition and understanding shock and sepsis.

This is an account of research and the reflections of a surgeon who enjoyed a busy practice and who did clinical along with basic research. Whether any of these contributions were relevant must be left to the judgment of others and the test of time. Some, I thought were important, and others, trivial. In this essay, I illustrate how certain efforts succeeded while others failed. Work was left undone and ideas remained unexplored in the hope that someone in the future might carry on and examine untested hypotheses. The rationale for basic research by clinicians includes curiosity, but mainly, the prospect that laboratory work can be translated into improved patient care. Most academic residencies and fellowships require research commitments from applicants usually to assist established faculty with ongoing projects. Some trainees view this opportunity with enthusiasm and others with cynicism, a necessary hurdle to clear before getting down to the practice of their specialty. Faculty surgeons must compete for grants, and national academic recognition is linked to peer-reviewed grant funding. A few surgeons who have pursued research as a sole occupation have become excellent physiologists or experimental pathologists.

MAKING EARS AND RUNNING A PUMP

As an intern, I saw a shy young boy, about nine years old, in the plastic surgery clinic at Columbia Presbyterian Hospital. He came into the examination room clutching a pull-on watch cap about his head. We sat face to face, as I had been taught to do with children. His mother stood silently by him, and I asked him what his problem was. For a long moment, the child did not respond. He silently removed his cap to show that he had no visible ears, just two small holes and vestigial skin tabs. The cap remained clutched tightly in his hands as he looked at me with pleading and vulnerable eyes. This encounter affected me deeply. Though I never found out what had been planned or done for him by Dr. Webster's Plastic Surgery Clinic, my first research project was an attempt to mold cartilage to reconstruct an external ear. Fashioning the complex shell-like helices and antihelices of the external human ear is a daunting surgical task. Attempts at ear reconstruction were, and remain, a difficult challenge for the art of plastic surgery. I considered stamping out a template of ear cartilage as if from a cookie cutter.

Dr. Richard B. Stark, a plastic surgeon at St. Luke's in New York, showed me an article by Dr. Lewis Thomas at the Rockefeller Institute, describing the remarkable effect of intravenous injection of the meat tenderizer, papain, into rabbits. Their ears wilted, producing floppy eared rabbits resembling cocker spaniels. We thought that we might be able to mold cartilage while it existed in this softened state. Dr. Stark offered laboratory resources to work on this problem during my second year of surgical training. At the same time, I worked with a group practicing the use of cardiopulmonary bypass on dogs prior to attempting a clinical open-heart case at St. Luke's Hospital.

I went downtown to see Dr. Thomas in his small cluttered office at the Rockefeller Institute. He shared practical details for the procedure and liked the prospect of putting his curious observation to possible practical use. We purchased papain, Seitz filters, and two dozen white New Zealand rabbits and we then injected the sterile, filtered papain solution intravenously into rabbits of varying ages. An overdose given into young rabbits would induce softening of tracheal cartilage and death due to tracheal ring collapse. As soft floppy ears appeared, we immediately stapled the wilted ears into unusual shapes, hoping to impose upon them a new and permanent structure. Cartilage softening was transient, and when the staples were removed after four to six weeks, the rabbits' ears sprang back to their original perky shapes. During this process, the normal blue staining of the cartilage matrix disappeared, to return when the ears had resumed their normal consistency. Cartilage apparently had an internal molecular or fibrous structure that mandated its unique form. With that conclusion, I left the project, as I had to fulfill my military obligation.

When I came back from the air force after three years, I found that Dr. Stark kept the work alive in the form of a poster.

At Stark's urging, I resumed these experiments. This time, I harvested cartilage and immersed the ear plates in ice-cold sterile saline. Overnight, these became soft and pliable while the ice-cold saline became opaque, seeming to extract a mucopolysaccharide from the cartilage matrix. This resulted in soft and malleable plates, probably viable, with the consistency of wet cardboard. Unique shapes could be achieved when the cartilage plate was molded and re-implanted into the abdominal wall of it original host. It seemed likely that the matrix, in some manner, helped cartilage maintain unique shapes. With special staining, we saw an orderly network of supporting connective tissue fibers, much like reinforcing struts within the cartilage matrix, which appeared unaltered by saline immersion.

We published these results in 1964, but the work did not lead to any clinical advances in cartilage molding or ear reconstruction. In 2002, Haisch, Klaring, and others from Berlin, commented that the cosmetic results of auricular reconstruction were still unsatisfactory. They described a tissue-engineering process using human nasal septal chondrocytes implanted within an ear-like cylinder. This process produced well-preserved auricular shapes and sizes in mice, but skin coverage and draping of these bioprostheses remain problematic. We still have much to learn about the structure and metabolism of cartilage as its deterioration in many individuals leads to disabling joint disease.

The practice of performing surgery on dogs with circulatory bypass and a bubble oxygenator was challenging and eventually rewarding. A nurse, Allegra Coons, a diener, Wilbur Smith, and I, created atrial cardiac defects for later repair using cardiopulmonary bypass. We learned tricks of blood balance and operative conduct to achieve satisfactory survival, and we also learned that we had to sit up all night with the dogs replacing blood and fluids while monitoring oxygenation and blood pressure. In 1958, we then ran the pump oxygenator for a successful open-heart case done in New York City by Drs.

Hugh Fitzpatrick and Peter Bossart when they closed an atrial septal defect in a young man. While open-heart procedures had been successful in Philadelphia, Minneapolis, and Houston, in New York hospitals, there had been, we were told, seventeen consecutive deaths after open-heart surgery. Just as we had done in the laboratory with our dogs, we sat up all night with this patient in an impromptu intensive care unit, set up across the cafeteria. My wife thought that I had been tending to another dog. We had learned about intensive care for postoperative patients. Modern intensive care units were established in the early 'sixties specifically to care for open-heart cases. Wilbur Smith remains in charge of cardiopulmonary bypass at St. Luke's Hospital, which continues to enjoy the excellent results of its pioneering heart program.

During the course of this work, we sacrificed dogs purchased from a local provider. I knew nothing about their provenance and we also used some dogs as blood donors. Since our goal was to achieve survival after two operations, we became attached to these animals and saw to it that they exercised on the roof and were well tended. It would have been impossible to develop heart surgery and vascular surgery without these sacrifices. Over the years, I have thought about these dogs and their contributions to surgical care. I remember one gratifying experience: a large affectionate German Shepherd with a fractured femur appeared in the laboratory to serve as a blood donor. A woman who lived on Park Avenue was his owner and had heard of our work. Her veterinarian had told her that there was nothing he could do and recommended euthanasia. St. Luke's had available the latest in orthopedic devices. Allegra Coons and I cleaned up the nasty fracture wound, gave penicillin and then placed an intramedullary nail we scavenged from the operating room. We continued intravenous antibiotics and a week later, returned this fine dog to a grateful lady. She made a donation to the laboratory and also insisted on paying me three hundred dollars, the first fee I ever received for a surgical procedure.

A PROSPECTIVE STUDY

Prospective randomized placebo-controlled trials have become a gold standard for evidence-based medicine. But, as we will see later, these are more difficult to use for testing operative interventions. We tested d-pantothenyl alcohol, a drug that was advertised as hastening bowel function after abdominal surgery. My fellow resident, Dr. William Reid, obtained a drug called Ilopan, which was donated by the maker, along with a supply of placebos. Drug and placebo were dispensed in either blue or red-labeled glass vials. We injected either drug or placebo after uncomplicated matched abdominal operations. The drug was given immediately postoperatively in the recovery room. To our surprise, whether we used drug or placebo, virtually all patients had bowel sounds. We had thought that the intestines became paralyzed immediately after surgery when, in fact, they were not. The observers first injecting this drug had heard bowel sounds immediately after operation and had been misled by uncontrolled observations. Few observers had ever listened in the immediate postoperative interval. The intestines tend to contract during the first hour or two after abdominal closure, and then, a period of inactivity follows.

But the residents all wanted their own patients to receive the drug rather than the placebo. Some of them managed to find out that the blue vials contained Ilopan while the red vials contained placebo. We took all the vials to our room to wipe off all the red and blue labeling with alcohol and acetone so we could continue to blind the study. We locked our call room securely, as some even tried to break our key for our coded cardboard boxes. Nurses and residents would search diligently for any remaining trace of color clinging to the glass vials. We concluded that bowel function returned when patients pass gas or feces. Individuals receiving drug or placebo required intravenous infusions for virtually equal-time intervals after operation. The functional endpoints of drug and placebo were exactly equal. Bowel sounds heard in the recovery room were a kind of red herring. We published these results, with no objections from the manufacturer of Ilopan, in the *American Journal of Surgery*. Over the years, I learned that presence or absence of postoperative bowel sounds means little, except with mechanical obstructions when these can become characteristically loud or when their sudden disappearance signals an intraabdominal catastrophe.

BILE AND GALLSTONES

In the fall of 1961, and through a frigid Ohio December, I worked for Dr. William D. Holden, the chief of surgery at Lakeside Hospital in Cleveland. He gave me time and resources to do research. I had access to new laboratories in the Wearn Research Building at Case Western Reserve. Perhaps I should have returned, once again, to the ear cartilage problem, but I had been considering the unique physico-chemical characteristics of bile after caring for a patient with a persistent biliary fistula. Fluids with low surface tension, such as bile, form fine droplets that could more easily leak from suture lines. I thought of measuring the surface tension of bile and comparing it to other bodily fluids. Surface activity of bile might relate to its ability to keep cholesterol in solution and, if not low enough, might lead to cholesterol precipitation and gallstones. Cholesterol had been named as "the sterol obtained from gallstones." The ability to solubilize fat should be reflected in the physico-chemical characteristics and surface tension measurement might yield clues about gallstone formation. Dogs rarely form gallstones and human cholesterol stones placed in the canine gallbladder bile dissolve, so I postulated that the surface tension of canine bile ought to be much lower than that of human bile.

Mr. J. R. Raines, professor of surgery at Charing Cross in London, had suggested in 1953 that abnormalities in the physico-chemical or micellar characteristics of bile salts led to gallstone formation. British surgeons are referred to as "Mister" rather than Doctor, as the Royal College of Physicians considered them descendants of barbers, but they are proud to be called "Mister."

Raines' novel hypothesis had attracted little attention or recognition. Micellar solubilization is a unique process that enhances lipid-holding capacity in admixtures of water and fats. These molecular colloid-like particles allow fats to dissolve in water. Thus, oil and water actually mix. Soaps are long-chain fatty acids that solubilize fat in the long-chain fatty part of the molecule, while charged particles face outward into the watery environment. Bile makes fat soluble for intestinal absorption much as soap removes fat along with dirt from skin.

A skilled Cleveland glass blower constructed an apparatus, to my specifications, to measure surface tension. Drop size and rate of formation could be precisely controlled with a micrometer burette. In a constant temperature room of 37 degrees Celsius, using control liquids of known surface tension, the method proved to be accurate to one-thousandth of a dyne. As predicted, the surface tension of canine gallbladder bile proved to be much lower than that of human gallbladder bile and, biochemically, canine bile exhibited a much higher bile acid content. As we diluted bile from patients with gallstones, inflections in the surface tension curves appeared, which did not occur in bile from normal gallbladders or dog bile. We suggested that this irregular behavior was due to disturbed micellar aggregation, as suggested by Mr. Raines. We also measured and compared the content of cholesterol, bile acids, and lecithin in human and gallbladder bile. Canine bile contained significantly more bile acid and much less cholesterol than human bile, while human bile had a higher content of cholesterol relative to bile acid and phospholipid content. We sent the manuscript to Dr. Loyal Davis, editor of *Surgery, Gynecology and Obstetrics,* who edited my manuscript with a blue pencil, with the admonition that, if I would accept simple declarative sentences, he would publish it. He advised omitting the biochemical tables. Drs. Small and Admirand in Boston later published elegant physicochemical studies to show that triangular coordinates of relative concentrations of cholesterol, bile acids and lecithin determined whether cholesterol would remain in solution. It seemed as if a cure for the dread scourge of gallstone disease was in sight.

But it was not to be that simple. We began analyzing human bile specimens collected from young healthy trauma cases without gallstones and found that bile cholesterol content almost always exceeded micellar limits set by Small and Admirand's triangular coordinates. These patients should have had stones, but did not. The Boston group suggested that this represented "pre-stone disease," i.e., all these people were destined to get stones based upon the triangular coordinates, but I thought that there must be other factors. The gallbladder concentrates bile from the liver some ten to fourteen times, so that not only abnormal relative concentrations of bile constituents, but also contraction and emptying of the gallbladder, affected the process of stone formation. Precipitated cholesterol particles might grow over repeated cycles of filling, intense concentration and incomplete expulsion of gallbladder contents.

In collaboration with two physical chemists, we examined a mathematical model postulating high water flux at the gallbladder wall. Our calculations showed large variations in solid concentrations due to the profound fluid flux as water was absorbed by the gallbladder wall, even predicting cholesterol precipitation within a wide and putatively normal range of cholesterol concentration relative to bile acid and lecithin. We published this work in the *Proceedings of the National Academy of Sciences*, but nothing more was ever heard about it.

Based on the biliary composition hypothesis, oral agents were created in hopes of favorably altering bile constituents to treat or prevent stones. However, these four decades of work have not influenced the prevalence of gallstones in Western society nor cured them medically. The bile acid, ursodeoxycholic acid, given by mouth, seemed initially to dissolve stones, but when the drug was stopped, gallstones recurred. In addition, the resulting smaller stones might more easily migrate into the common duct draining the liver, causing a more serious problem than if they had been confined to the gallbladder. Lithotripsy, breaking up stones with shock waves, did not prove as effective as for kidney stones. Gallstones tend to form during periods of rapid weight loss, but in recent controlled trials (*Journal of Surgical Research 2002* and *Alimentary Pharmacology and Therapeutics, 2000*), neither ursodeoxycholic acid nor agents promoting gallbladder motility reduced the rate of gallstone formation with weight loss. The gallstone problem remains essentially unsolved.

We now use a surgical laparoscopic technique to remove gallbladders containing stones. Surgeons in Georgia and in France pioneered this minimally invasive approach, over the howls of academicians, and after battalions of investigators had worked on the gallstone problem with unprepossessing results. But interesting lessons were learned. During fasting, weight loss, or prolonged intravenous nutrition, cholesterol excretion and failure of gallbladder contraction probably both cause gallstones.

Gertrude Stein once said, "A difference to be difference must make a difference." Gallstone research, overall, has not, as yet, amounted to much. We still need surgery to treat gallstone disease. I thought, early on, that this was an interesting problem, but an internal reviewer and critic at Western Reserve indicted our gallstone research problem as "pedestrian." It was true that little romance or glamour seemed to reside in gallstones. However, thinking about cholesterol and bile acid metabolism led me into research on atherosclerosis, which did have a certain cachet. In a sense, atherosclerosis might be the flip side of gallstone disease. Cholesterol gallstones likely represent an attempt of the body to rid itself of excess lipid. Both diseases are common in Western cultures.

During this work, I encountered the harsh politics of science. We had submitted an abstract, *The Micellar Nature of Bile*, to an American Medical Association Forum in New York City. Dr. Franz Inglefinger, gastroenterologist and editor, of the prestigious *New England Journal of Medicine*, presided grumpily over a poorly attended session in a stuffy room at a Holiday Inn on Manhattan's West Side. When I finished the presentation, no comments or questions came from him or the audience. Actually, he seemed decidedly unhappy with my presentation. We had been instructed to deliver the manuscript to a session moderator, but Dr. Inglefinger was quite reluctant to accept the manuscript. As he hastily departed, I shoved it into his hands.

DECEPTION AND DIARRHEA

I was jubilant about the opportunity to present this work, but I overestimated the importance of my rudimentary physico-chemical insights and, also, of the occasion. Eve and I drove to New York City with our son Larry, then three years old. We visited relatives and I reconnected with some friends in the Chinese community. We had real bird's nest soup in Chinatown. Our journey home to Cleveland was painful and slow. We developed severe diarrhea, chills and fever en route. Our stool culture showed positive for salmonella and the three of us required long courses of tetracycline.

After our return, I heard nothing about our submission for months, and then I called the AMA editors. The paper conveyed to Inglefinger had not been transmitted to them. I sent a revised copy, which was published promptly in the *Journal of the American Medical Association*. I learned that Inglefinger's department in Boston had a group working on the physico-chemical characteristics of bile. These workers proved later to be my friends, Drs. Small and Admirand. Their contributions on bile composition were deservedly well funded, but they never considered the gallbladder contraction hypothesis to be important. Soon after the *JAMA* article appeared, a senior thoracic surgeon at Western Reserve commented that this kind of work was useless. I continue to worry that he might have been right.

LOWERING CHOLESTEROL: MAKING A DIFFERENCE

Studies of biliary dynamics did not prove to be a complete loss. We observed that common bile duct drainage, something routinely done after common duct surgery, drastically lowered serum cholesterol. This observation yielded a tool to see whether arrest or regression of experimental atherosclerosis might occur in response to lowered serum cholesterol. Biliary diversion gave us means of seeing if plaques, at various stages of development, might regress or stabilize when blood cholesterol fell. We proved in animals that plaque regression and arrest occurred when blood cholesterol was sufficiently lowered. Dr. Henry Buchwald used ileal bypass clinically to create bile acid and cholesterol loss in patients with high cholesterol and heart disease. He demonstrated fewer heart attacks or need for vascular surgery in these individuals but no prolongation of life. I did some of these operations, but the resulting diarrhea appeared unacceptable to some of my patients.

Our first paper was published in 1967 in *The Surgical Forum*, a venue for young surgeons. From 1967 to 1969, Drs. William Insull Jr., Charles A. Hubay, and laboratory associates, Annie Robinson and Paul Hartman, and I contributed a series of studies on bile acid secretion, biliary diversion, and the relationship of serum cholesterol to progression and regression of experimental atherosclerosis. Dr. William Insull Jr. provided editorial and scientific discipline.

We began by using dogs as an experimental model for atherosclerosis. We ablated thyroid gland function with radioactive iodine, a diet containing cholesterol, bile acids and a drug, thiouracil. Fortunately, this model proved to be quite robust, and the dogs were easy to manage. We surgically short circuited the biliary tract by diverting bile toward the end of the intestine. This procedure, combined with a return to normal diet, dramatically lowered serum cholesterol levels. We could then open the aorta to see plaques whiten and shrink, carefully repairing the artery for serial observations and examining other sites as well. We found that cholesterol levels approximating 150mg/dl cholesterol were required for consistent plaque regression. Concurrent serial arteriograms in the animals also showed less lumen intrusion as plaques regressed.

At the time, we documented arteriographic regression over intervals of eighteen months in two patients whose cholesterol was reduced below 150 mg/dl. But there was still a long way to go. It was difficult to convince consultants, mainly pathologists on the grant review committees at the National Institutes of Health, of the practicality of atherosclerotic plaque regression or control in man. Some regarded human disease an inevitable consequence of aging; experimental work on regression in animal models was suspect. Many investigators had worked previously with rabbits, and these animals show disease progression even with reversion to a low-cholesterol diet. In rabbits, considerable lipid remained in the liver and spleen so that when the atherogenic diet was stopped, elevated lipid levels persisted and disease increased in severity. We found progression in hypothyroid dogs followed for several years with total cholesterol levels as low as 235mg/dl. These dogs developed both aneurysmal and occlusive lesions. A threshold cholesterol level existed above which atherosclerosis progressed, and this level was not very high. But at that time, a cholesterol level of 300mg/dl was accepted as normal for humans.

Dr. Gardiner McMillan at the National Institutes of Health had done some of the early rabbit experiments. But he was open-minded enough to spend a great deal of time helping me formulate acceptable grant applications. The hypotheses, he said, must be supported by "more than just a pious wish." Our canine model of atherosclerosis did not satisfy everyone. The NIH stimulated development of subhuman primate models of atherosclerosis, believing that these would more closely approximate human disease. Actually, the advanced lesions of the hypothyroid dogs appeared to me to accurately mimic human lesions, producing similar complications, including stroke, myocardial infarction and aneurysms. Occlusive disease in the distal aorta of dogs sometimes caused gangrene of the tail. Still, the use of monkeys seemed to catch on and the subhuman primate became a common model for study of atherosclerosis.

We obtained a local Heart Association grant to feed a colony of rhesus monkeys in Luray, Virginia, with massive concentrations of lard and cholesterol along with conventional monkey chow. These monkeys became obese and developed modest arterial fatty streaks that were not as severe as plaques seen in our dogs or in humans. With a change of the experimental diet to cakes containing eggs, corn syrup, and sugar with only .5% cholesterol by weight, serum cholesterol in the monkeys increased to 600 mg/dl. Atheromatous disease rapidly developed. The cakes were yellow and quite tasty, much like ordinary baked goods, and the laboratory staff once served them, with chocolate icing, during vascular grand rounds at Lakeside Hospital. This created a minor sensation, but clearly, these cakes were probably no worse than ordinary doughnuts. One Christmas morning, I was making homemade doughnuts on a device that I had been given as a gift. While adding ingredients, I suddenly realized that I was recreating our atherogenic monkey diet.

With the return to a normal diet, angiography and direct surgical observations in monkeys also showed plaque regression. Intermediate fibrofatty plaques regressed and collagen content or scar tissue sometimes decreased and sometimes increased in certain arterial sites. Early lesions were largely symmetrical, though for some reason that I could never completely grasp, more advanced lesions tended to be asymmetrical, and never became as severe as those observed in our dogs. Dr. Mark Armstrong and associates at the University of Iowa published the first primate observations of regression using comparative autopsy studies. They felt that collagen or scar tissue eventually decreased in the lesions, an observation that our group working with Dr. Leroy Klein did not confirm. We found that scar tissue in some sites tended to increase during regression. Actually, a local increase in scar tissue and a decrease in cholesterol would be favorable for stabilizing plaques. The animal experiments performed from 1967 through 1974, along with a review of the epidemiology of atherosclerosis, motivated us to monitor and to try to control elevated lipid levels in patients with vascular disease.

We aimed to achieve serum cholesterol levels below 200mg/dl, and later, total cholesterol levels below 150mg/dl with LDL cholesterol levels below 100 mg/dl. After three decades, most agree that these levels are needed for patients with vascular disease and for those who have other associated risk factors. Coronary and vascular diseases remain as our most common causes of death. Thousands of papers on atherosclerosis are published each year. We began screening vascular patients in 1966, advising dietary alterations when lipids were high, but we found abnormal lipid levels in only one-third of our patients with established disease. Our diet recommended reduction of saturated fat intake and red meat, avoiding canned processed meats and all dairy products including butter and eggs, and importantly, no added sugar. We erred in advising margarine as a substitute for butter. Margarine was later found to have a harmful trans fatty acid. We were possibly too harsh about eggs, but these, along with sugar, were important constituents of our atherogenic monkey cakes. Dietary controversy persists and, with a few exceptions, the lipid response to our diet proved quite modest.

At that time, the only medication available to lower cholesterol was a powder, the bile acid sequestrant cholestyramine. When we added cholestyramine to monkey cakes, we found the drug effective in lowering cholesterol and improving plaques. But cholestyramine proved to be constipating in man and most patients hated to take it. In advanced disease and in sick patients, hyperlipidemia was often absent even while vascular complications progressed. In my own and in Dr. DeBakey's large series of vascular patients in the sixth and seventh decades, total cholesterol levels ranged from 165-170mg/dl. Other factors appeared to promote disease progression and complications, and lipid control was not the complete answer.

Genetics determine lipid metabolism in different individuals and species. People with a congenital defect in internalizing their low-density lipoprotein cholesterol into liver cells have difficulty converting low-density lipoprotein (LDL) cholesterol into bile acid. In some unusual cases, when the genes promoting this defect are paired or homozygous, serum cholesterol rises to above 600 mg/ml and death occurs by age thirty. This condition, familial hypercholesterolemia, can also cause intermediate lipid elevations when the genetics are heterozygous, that is, only one gene exists. In these cases, about one in five or six hundred live births, cholesterol levels are set at about 300mg/dl and, in untreated cases, death begins to occur by the fifth decade. Brown and Goldstein won a Nobel Prize for their work defining the role of hepatic LDL receptors in regulating blood cholesterol levels. They commented that, while hypercholesterolemia was crucial, its exact effects on the arterial wall were poorly defined. Elevated lipid levels alone, as important as they may be, cannot account for all cases of complications such as heart attack, aneurysm and stroke. Immune and inflammatory responses also modulate disease severity. Local and systemic responses vary considerably between individual humans and subhuman primates such as rhesus, cynamolgus, and stump-tailed macaques. Species differences are important. In Luray, we found a colony of skunks eating atherogenic diets in the sheds housing our rhesus monkeys. In what became a truly odiferous experience, Dr. Ted Roth, a veterinarian, shot two of them, contending he could do this before they emitted their protective aroma. Roth, of course, failed. Once we got past the smell, we found their arterial systems to be pristine. Another variable, "beyond cholesterol" in Dr. David Steinberg's words, is oxidation of low-density lipoprotein cholesterol, which makes the lipid proinflammatory and induces foam cell formation, the first step in forming an atherosclerotic plaque. Lately, experimental data using immunologically activated cells may controvert this hypothesis. Unfortunately, clinical trials using antioxidants such as vitamins C and E have not reduced death due to coronary disease.

As a result of clinical observations and experimental work in atherosclerosis, I began to recognize differing patterns, severity and rates of disease progression. Plaques ranged from unstable soft, oatmeal-like yellow lesions (atheroma, or porridge-like) to stable fibrotic or calcified lesions (sclerosis or scarring). This is important as different stages and distributions of atherosclerosis may require different medical or surgical approaches. The diversity of this disease is such that Drs. DeBakey and McMillan both felt that atheroscerosis might not be one entity, but rather, related families of differing clinicopathologic entities. I am still not sure, but as

Dr. DeBakey recently commented, "Everything about atherosclerosis is controversial." I am more comfortable with a unified or simplified hypotheses—Occam's razor—and prefer to consider atherogenesis as a single process.

It is worthwhile to consider atherosclerosis from an epidemiologic standpoint. During infancy at vulnerable sites within arteries, worldwide and in all populations, a minute core of cholesterol in foam cells and a few inflammatory cells accumulate during infancy. When total serum cholesterol in the population does not exceed 150 mg/dl, this process appears to be of little consequence and atherosclerosis is virtually absent. In Western industrial cultures, fatty streaks in the arteries progress to complex plaques that calcify and ulcerate, and acquire friable scar tissue, superimposed clot and collections of inflammatory cells. The superimposition of clot or ruptures of plaques are the mechanisms leading to heart attack, stroke and limb loss.

While sick or elderly atherosclerotics often exhibit low lipid levels, these individuals, if they are not diabetic, usually will have had past intense exposures, including lipid abnormalities, hypertension, or smoking. Irrespective of lipid control, smoking cessation is critically important in determining clinical outcomes. Powerful drugs acting on hepatic metabolism can effectively reduce serum lipids as well as the inflammatory response, and cut heart attack rates. Inflammatory processes cause disease progression and smoking appears to promote these processes through some mechanism as yet poorly understood.

In 1970, we published clinical guidelines for treatment of surgical patients with atherosclerosis and hyperlipidemia in *Surgery, Gynecology and Obstetrics*. *New England Journal of Medicine* reviewers, six months earlier, stated that we presented insufficient evidence to support this view. We thought that surgeons should contribute to preventative measures and systemic treatment based on our clinical and laboratory experiences. Some thought this nonsense; surgeons ought to be concerned with and confined to surgical matters. The medical establishment took three decades to reach a consensus and to accept the idea that hyperlipdemia is associated with increased risk of developing atherosclerosis and its complications. Now, everyone is supposed to know their cholesterol number and TV advertisements show little children serving their parents heart-healthy Cheerios in bed. This is at once gratifying but also disturbing, as Cheerios might not be the whole answer.

Based on data showing that aortic graft occlusion was related to continued smoking, Dr. Hubay and I, in 1970, suggested removing cigarette machines from Lakeside Hospital. This suggestion infuriated staff physicians and our chief of staff, who was a smoker. I confess that I still like to smoke an occasional cigar and I would resent being forced to stop this practice. Now, all hospitals are smoke-free; I smoke cigars in my car. Smoking is an independent risk factor causing coronary and vascular disease, though in countries like China and Japan, where lipid levels are low, smoking is not tightly associated with atherosclerosis, as in Western society. Cessation of smoking can avert the need for surgery, and in examining disease progression, the onset of vascular complications occurs a decade earlier in smokers, and earlier in men than in women. Women seem to have more difficulty with smoking cessation than men. Cessation of cigarette smoking is also critical for the durability of vascular reconstructions of all types. The deleterious effects of smoking on atherosclerosis and after surgical interventions have been confirmed and reconfirmed many times over. Smokers should not have elective operations for vascular disease unless they can get help with smoking cessation. Graft occlusion and repeated operations cause a much worse situation than if the arteries had remained undisturbed. Vascular services still need to develop formal antismoking treatment programs. As yet, few clinics offer this service in a systematic manner.

ASPIRIN AND ANTIPLATELET AGENTS

We began to assay the effects of aspirin and dipyridamole on atherosclerosis upon our colony of rhesus monkeys in the late 1970s. The desirability of lipid interventions, I thought, was settled, but motivating people to accept dietary changes proved difficult. I found it easier to have patients accept major surgery than to influence them or their family to change dietary habits. The few that followed dietary advice did so with good effect, but overall cholesterol reduction was only about 10-12%, which failed to meet threshold reduction criteria to actually effect favorable arterial changes. I thought it might be more practical to take pills that would interfere with the disease process. The results were surprising and paradoxical. The doses of aspirin and dipyrimadole, then prescribed for human use, made atheromatous disease progress more rapidly in rhesus monkeys. We now began to see, for the first time, arterial occlusion in rhesus monkeys receiving the drugs. In injured rabbit arteries, we found that this drug combination retarded healing so that the final result was more arterial thickening.

The daily recommended dose of aspirin has been reduced progressively from four tablets to one aspirin tablet, 325 mg. Some suggest that 81 mg, a baby aspirin, is sufficient. The American Heart Association recommends aspirin dosages ranging from 60 to over 100 mg. We have yet to delineate optimal doses and efficacy of various types of antiplatelet drugs. We still do not know the proper dose of aspirin and the establishment recommendations remain confusing. A regular aspirin tablet taken daily reduces the occurrence of heart attacks and in an acute situations, reduces mortality, but the penalty is an increased rate of bleeding and hemorrhagic stroke in some subsets of patients. I continue to take a baby aspirin, 81mg, every day or two, and recommend this for my patients.

SHOCK

Shock research at Western Reserve Surgery had a long-standing history, beginning with Dr. George Crile's work the early 1900s. The causes of inadequate tissue perfusion or shock are multiple. In surgical patients, the main causes of shock are blood and fluid loss and infection. Shock, derived from the French "choc," had long been a mysterious entity. A French military surgeon, Henri Françoise LeDran, coined the term after seeing what happened when armored knights first met blunt injuries in battle. As far back as the Battle of Troy, military surgeons understood penetrating injuries and their outcomes. But diffuse internal injuries, by and large, awaited the explosive force of gunpowder. The picture of shock—pallor with a rapid heartbeat and circulatory failure in the absence of visible penetrating injuries—appeared mysterious. Dr. George Crile Sr., in Cleveland early in the twentieth century, alluded to the death of a young man following a femoral fracture as "a rude unhinging of the machinery of life." The young man had been injured in a trolley car accident, and when first admitted, appeared stable and had been joking with his attendants. What he and his contemporaries did not know at that time was that the death of his young patient had been caused by hidden hemorrhage and fluid loss incident to major fractures. Dr. Alfred Blalock of Johns Hopkins demonstrated this hidden fluid loss two decades later using experimental injury in a dog model. Years later, at Western Reserve, we saw, or thought we saw, with an electron microscope, the basis of Crile's "rude unhinging," hidden within the cells of shocked animals.

Carl Wiggers, a professor of physiology, had developed animal models of hemorrhagic shock showing the existence of a point of no return or "irreversible shock" in spite of blood replacement. The cause of this irreversible state was unknown. Dr. William Drucker, adapting the Wiggers' model to rats, had demonstrated the metabolic effects of shock with an initial hyperglycemia and late hypoglycemia and lactic acid production which suggested failure of energy production. Drs. John Davis and Thomas Krizek studied the distinct shock-inducing pathways of gram-negative and gram-positive bacteria, while Drs. Donald Gann and Hastings K. Wright delineated the many neuroendocrine effects of shock.

When the Lions Club of Cleveland donated an EMU-3 RCA electron microscope to the department, Dr. Holden suggested that we investigate the ultrastructural abnormalities in hemorrhage and endotoxemia. The availability of this powerful instrument was like having the first telescope to examine the heavens. But first, we had to cut ultra-fine tissue sections with a glass knife, fix and embed these tissue slices and obtain high-resolution photographs. At first, we wasted a good deal of time having to learn this process. When we finally got reasonable pictures, although not as good as I might have wished, we saw striking ultra-structural cellular changes in hemorrhagic shock not visible by ordinary light microscopy. The shape of mitochondria, key energy-generating organelles, changed from oblong to spherical. The cells became swollen with fluid, the endoplasmic reticulum or protein manufacturing apparatus was distorted, and the lysosomes, so-called suicide packets, appeared enlarged and increased in numbers. The ordinarily fine nuclear chromatin clumped in a random fashion, presaging the process we now call programmed cell death. Yet, the cells were not dead. Just as in examining the heavens with a powerful telescope, there was an inordinate amount to see at the cellular level.

The distortion of mitochondria was particularly interesting given what had been learned of the physiology of shock. Morphologic alterations in these unique organelles seemed logically related to the metabolic change from aerobic to anaerobic metabolism during shock, and the increasing oxygen uptake, with accumulation of lactic and other acids in the bloodstream. We isolated the mitochondria to study their energy-generating function and respiration and found that isolated mitochondria from shocked animals showed deranged function. Their oxygen uptake in resting states was sluggish. Energy production—when we added a substrate as fuel—was impaired and poorly coupled to oxygen uptake. Energy generation had become quite inefficient. After adequate fluid treatment, mitochondrial isolates from treated animals returned to normal. These observations appeared important, but I could not think of a way, other than adequate fluid treatment, to intervene at this level, to treat or prevent shock. I read all I could about mitochondria. This became lonely work as my surgical friends kidded me, "What are you doing, Ralph? Can you cut them with a knife?" But I could not or would not, at the time, give up on mitochondria, even as some of our residents urged me back into the operating room.

We used Ducker's rat shock model to estimate optimal fluid replacement based on its standard mortality and, at the same time, I tried to quantify cellular edema and distortion and intracellular fluid shift. As shown by Dr. G. Tom Shires and his Dallas group, we confirmed that treatment of hemorrhagic shock models with crystalloid salt solutions, as opposed to blood alone, produced the best survival and the best-looking cells.

Alignment of the double condenser microscope had initially posed a serious problem. I visited RCA in Camden, New Jersey, to learn how to do this. We abolished the Ajax scrubbing routine promulgated by one of our technicians. Dr. Holden enjoyed smoking cigars in the laboratory, annoying our technician who became more and more truculent. I guess that he wanted her to leave, so with a mischievous gleam in his eye, he would hand me a cigar to smoke each time I left our office suite for the laboratory. I had quit smoking cigarettes as a resident, but I began smoking cigars during those years at Western Reserve. My wife blames Dr. Holden for this, but I like them, and I am careful about where and when I do smoke. When this technician left for another laboratory, smoked out as it were, we hired a talented young African American, Mr. John Wilburn, who proved to be an enormous asset to our research efforts. He helped move the laboratory to the University of Nevada School of Medicine in 1979, and John's talent and patience made much of our work possible.

SHOCK: BOXES WITHIN BOXES

For more than a decade, we had grant funding to study shock and atherosclerosis. I was intrigued with the cell biology and the morphology revealed by the electron microscope and simultaneously driven by the immediate clinical challenges of vascular disease. During this time, I was elected president of the Electron Microscopy Society and I discussed this dilemma with Dr. George Palade, a visiting scientist from the Rockefeller Institute. He told me that I should persist; a surgeon might best address surgical issues in basic science. But I felt quite inadequate to do the task. One of my young associates joked that, "It is better to be a dilettante than a bore." Neither is desirable, but because general surgery is such a wide field, I, like many in this discipline, tended to seek out, and even welcome, diverse challenges. Each of these efforts took on a life of its own, separated from day-to-day clinical life. I needed to come to terms with the fact that I was doing too much and not doing it as well as I could.

I came to fully grasp the complexity of mitochondria, and the more I focused on them, the more complex I found them to be. References to mitochondria in the *Current Contents* grew to more than I could scan. In trying to influence the lethal course of hemorrhage and, later, the effects of gram-negative infections or endotoxemia, I came to believe, perhaps too tenaciously, that mitochondria were a key to this problem. I reached out to a brilliant mitochondrial scientist, Dr. Lena Mela, at the University of Pennsylvania, who had been trained in Britain Chance's laboratories. We had both shown that mitochondrial respiration and energy production were disrupted by endotoxemia, but we could not understand how the large endotoxin molecule could enter cells. After a while, Lena came to believe that the main problem in shock resided within cell membranes and related to calcium fluxes rather than to failure of mitochondrial energy production. Her interests turned toward brain hypoxia. I became discouraged with this line of research as we had yet to do more than describe phenomena.

We did see that intestinal barrier function became compromised in late hemorrhagic shock and this breach allowed endotoxin to enter the bloodstream, accounting for the similar ultrastructural abnormalities between late hemorrhage and endotoxemia. Dr.

Robert Rhodes then showed that the loss of the intestinal barrier function correlated temporally with the onset of hepatic mitochondrial malfunction. Dr. Jacob Fine of Boston, many years before, had demonstrated endotoxin in the blood in shock using a *Limulus* assay, and we could confirm that rising *Limulus* titers correlated with loss of the intestinal barrier and onset of mitochondrial dysfunction. Scientists can devote entire careers to endlessly probing an interaction such as this, publish interesting papers, get grants and become professors. Ultimately, I came to believe that I was contributing nothing other than phenomenological description. I could not find my way completely out of the shock studies with a tangible intervention strategy. Late shock causes multiple organ failure (MOF), and the more recently recognized, a systemic inflammatory response syndrome (SIRS). Naming and describing these processes has given us important insights, but we have yet to provide specific interventions at a cellular level. Naming these processes does provide taxonomy as a first step in the solution of this problem.

I had hoped that we could create "super mitochondria," which would resist hypoxia, ischemia, and infectious assault. In a curious experimental model that attracted little attention after its publication in *Diabetes*, we did come close to this goal. Dr. Yutaka Harano, now professor of medicine in Osaka, and I found that diabetic rats developed greatly enlarged hepatic mitochondria. These contained more protein and metabolized fatty substrates more efficiently than mitochondria from livers of normal animals. Work in Dr. John Davis' laboratory by Dr. Tom Krizek showed that these same diabetic rats, paradoxically, resisted the lethal effects of endotoxemia. Somehow, mitochondrial ability to metabolize fatty acids and other substrates related to endotoxin resistance. But, we did not get much further with this finding.

We also thought that factors causing organ failure in late shock might be prevented by some kind of pretreatment. Steroids achieve this if given before an endotoxic insult. But how can one predetermine this? We wondered if mitochondria alone generate the enormous energy needed to maintain cellular membrane gradients, or is this more an intrinsic property of cell membranes? Later investigators questioned the significance of mitochondria in shock. I believe some investigators did this prematurely, as many of the isolated control mitochondrial isolates from other surgical laboratories functioned, in my opinion, unacceptably by basic science standards. Their isolates were sick to start with. I may have been a dilettante, but Paul Hartman and Annie Robinson in our laboratory worked to achieve tightly coupled control isolates to compare with those obtained from shocked animals, so these changes were quite significant, and reproduced in Dr. Mela's laboratory.

Cytokines are products of activated round cells. These proteins and their receptors are now under intense study in shock and other disease states. I initially labored under the misapprehension that systemic cytokine changes were epiphenomena of advanced processes rather than themselves, in some manner, etiologic. Many cytokines exist, have opposing actions and are hard to quantify in blood and tissues. Endotoxemia stimulates cytokine production and the entry of these messengers into cells likely accounts for the intracellular effects of endotoxin we could not understand. I had expressed reservations about cytokine studies to enthusiastic young surgical investigators, and will have to eat my words.

I tested the endotoxin hypothesis clinically during aortic reconstructive surgery. Alternate patients received a rigorous bowel preparation including antibiotics, and others received a single preoperative enema. Blood endotoxin levels in each group were tested by *Limulus* assay at key intervals during the procedure. I postulated that the blood endotoxin levels would correlate with release of aortic clamps, drops in blood pressure, and overall blood loss. Instead, endotoxin levels surged just at the start of surgery, when we manipulated and retracted the intestines. Bowel preparation had no influence on the time course or severity of endotoxemia. I never published this work; at the time, I could not understand these results. But I now understand the reason that minimally invasive procedures or extraperitoneal approaches are so benign.

After fifteen years of work, we had reams descriptive data. But we were still documenting rather than influencing the clinical course of shock. For example, in endotoxic shock, fibrin deposits could be seen in all the small vessels of vital organs. Treatment with heparin abolished the fibrin deposits but did not alter the lethal course of endotoxemia. For a while, some clinicians even gave heparin to patients in shock, which made them bleed. I envisioned a lifetime of probing into smaller and more complicated boxes in these animal models. The research of Dr. G. Tom Shires had already made a difference in treatment. He showed that the cellular edema with the intracellular sequestration of fluid correlated with loss of cell membrane potential, and advised, over traditional objections, the use of crystalloid salt solutions to compensate for intracellular fluid translocation. This concept yielded quantitative improvements in shock management with one exception: Patients with massive bleeding, for example, in ruptured aortic aneurysms, need clamping of the vessel and control of bleeding before crystalloid salt solution or blood to raise blood pressure. Excess crystalloid given in the field or in emergency rooms by over-zealous resuscitation before surgery caused thin blood that did not clot, the so-called red-ink syndrome. Mortality from ruptured aneurysms increased from 40 to 80% during this time. In these cases, a developing and enthusiastic emergency medical network contributed, unwittingly, to a higher mortality for ruptured aneurysms by trying to raise blood pressure with fluid administration before operative interventions.

The emergency room staff at George Washington graciously asked me to speak on "Emergency Room Management and Resuscitation of Ruptured Aneurysms." I showed a blank slide; there was none. The patient needed, I told them, a clamp on the aorta. Attempts to raise blood pressure before this were inadvisable. This caveat aside, from the start, Shires was way ahead in this field. Our work did not uncover a magic bullet to treat cellular dysfunction. Dr. Holden felt that the shock research was more promising than our atherosclerosis research. Some clinical actions and guidelines, based on observational insights, did prove relevant.

Drs. Byron McGregor and Richard Bomberger in Reno showed that moderate fluid replacement after aortic surgery closely approximated Shire's predictions of intracellular fluid loss. Patients need adequate and not excessive resuscitation, and, as pointed out by Dr. H. Treat Cafferata, "a second hit" must be anticipated and avoided. But I still wonder if cells might be conditioned to resist the effects of shock until resuscitation can be achieved.

SEX AND THE SURGEON

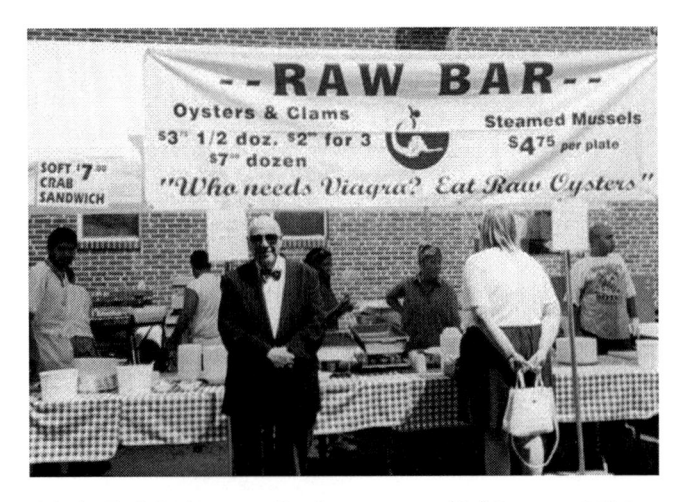

Little Italy's Answer for impotence, Baltimore, 2001

In the spring of 1974, I operated on a forty-eight-year-old Ohioan farmer with aortoiliac occlusive disease. His leg pain limited his farm work. He had high serum cholesterol, lived at home with his mother, evinced little interest in women, and mentioned, quite in passing, that he was impotent. The blockages consisted of relatively soft atheroma involving the distal aorta, common iliac arteries, and extending a short way into the internal iliac or pelvic arteries on both sides. Endarterectomy restored blood flow into the pelvic vessels as well as to the lower limbs. The procedure was done so that the genital nerves remained undisturbed. A book by our former professor of anatomy at New York University, Dr. Joseph Pick, helped with this dissection. One of the farmer's seemingly minor complaints had been erectile dysfunction. Four days postoperatively, he called me to his bedside and confided with some distress, "I am in trouble, Doc." The appearance of an attractive nurse had engendered a spontaneous erection. He moved out of his mother's house and later married. This clinical experience led me into the interesting field of erectile dysfunction and its diagnosis and treatment.

I described this experience to Dr. Lester Persky, the chief urologist at Case Western Reserve, "Lester, this might seem like a trivial observation, but this man has regained normal erections." Lester looked thoughtful and replied, "Ralph, this is very important. Impotence is a devastating complaint." Dr. Persky and his associate, Dr. Kalish Kedia, as well as other urologists, became key collaborators in this work. At the first conference on "Corpus Cavernosum Revascularization," convened by Dr. Adrian Zorgniotti at NYU in 1979, I presented methods of large vessel reconstruction. The consensus at that time was that poor penile arterial flow associated with aging caused erectile dysfunction, so direct penile revascularization attracted considerable attention. Later work showed that failure of penile smooth muscle relaxation is the most common mechanism in erectile dysfunction. My descriptions of operative techniques for large vessels and case selection generated widespread interest and invitations to lecture. I had been fortunate to encounter that first patient in that time and in that place.

Dr. Steven Levine, professor of psychiatry at Case Western Reserve, first recognized that many cases of impotence were organic rather than psychogenic in origin. He referred some of our patients with arteriogenic impotence. When I asked Steven how he was able to differentiate psychogenic from organic impotence, he replied, "Ralph, this is my business." Levine's historical criteria that differentiate organic from psychogenic impotence remain a helpful and first-line tool for patient assessment. Colleagues in Cleveland, Ohio, Reno, Nevada, and Washington, D.C., helped me evaluate the efficacy of vascular surgery, which was better for large vessel reconstruction than for microvascular bypasses. Donna Stouffer Kowallek, a clinical vascular nurse specialist at the Reno VAMC, used penile blood pressure and pulse volume recordings to characterize patients with arteriogenic impotence. These objective measurements provided a useful guide to dosage of intracavernous injection agents and evaluating the patency of bypass procedures. Normal pulse waves correlated closely with bypass success and restoration of normal function. Dr. Tom Lue of San Francisco later used ultrasound evaluation after intracavernous injection to assess penile flow, and this procedure became the focus of testing by urologists specializing in erectile dysfunction. Invasive diagnosis and surgery are now less frequently needed as effective medications to induce penile muscle relaxation have become available.

The fascinating thing about the first aortoiliac operation in 1974 was that, at the same time, Dr. Vaclav Michal of Prague, Czechoslovakia, made the same observation after performing a similar procedure. His papers appeared in the Czech and Russian literature and we later became friends. Dr. Ronald Virag, a vascular surgeon in Paris, began to explore variants of microvascular bypasses. More importantly, Virag observed that intracavernous injection of papaverine caused erection. Virag's 1982 observations, along with those of Brindley, who publicly self-injected phentolamine, an alpha-blocking agent, provided the means for diagnosis and of treatment. Intracavernous injection, billed as the four-hour erection, found its way into *Playboy*. Dr. Virag was outraged by the resulting spectacular publicity. Sex sells but keeping treatment for sexual dysfunction within ethical bounds remains a challenge. Penile injection remains effective treatment when oral agents fail, but self-injection must be done with caution and with judicious patient education. Prolonged and painful involuntary erections occur with improper use and this may lead to irreversible scarring in the delicate penile tissues. This took a while to learn, and for some time, we had to treat such self-induced priapism, often late at night in emergency rooms.

After screening and treating over one thousand men complaining of impotence, we reported in 1990 that only about 7% of men with erectile dysfunction were candidates for vascular procedures after they failed to respond to medical or injection treatment. The major focus of vascular procedures evolved to become a means for the prevention of erectile dysfunction after aortic interventions, and, in younger patients, restoration of blood flow after trauma. This work yielded some of my most grateful patients. Unexpected results occurred in three women. Women rarely complain of sexual dysfunction, and these patients, all in their mid-forties, required aortic surgery. I used exactly the same techniques I had employed in men, preserving the pelvic nerves and ensuring blood flow into the pelvic arteries as well as to the lower extremities. Two women thanked me profusely, not for relief of leg symptoms, but for other benefits. One gave up seeing her psychiatrist who had been treating her for orgasmic failure; the second was relieved of vaginal dryness and dyspareunia. The third woman became overtly seductive, and ultimately ran away with one of her husband's friends. Differences in arousal and function between sexes has been likened to the difference between a light switch in men, on and off, and, and in women, a complex set of high fidelity equipment. But both sexes need adequate blood flow and intact neural arcs. In men, visual erotic stimulation (VES) using pornographic tapes can be used to incite a visible erection that can be measured, gauged, and tested. Response testing in women relies on vaginal lubrication, which is more difficult to observe or measure. Urologists working in the area are now exploring other measures of female arousal and function. I never used VES to assess sexual dysfunction. Ordinary pornographic films seemed to be in poor taste for a consulting room and I could only imagine what the *Washington Post* might say. I questioned a lady coworker who was studying female arousal using VES. I said that I had thought that women did not like pornography. Her reply was, "How do you know?" I learned that I knew less and less every day.

A generation of scientific urologists including Rajfer, Goldstein, Lue, Lewis, Padma-Natha, Adaiken and others, advanced our knowledge of penile smooth muscle physiology in many important ways. The baton passed from vascular surgeons to urologists, and deservedly so, as a result of their scientific efforts. I once reminded an audience of urologists that, at the end of every aorta, there dangles a penis, hoping to emphasize their need to search for large vessel disease among their patients. My statement was followed by laughter. I was quickly corrected. In half of the cases, there will be a clitoris. About two-thirds of men are now treated successfully with medication, sildenafil, which inhibits the breakdown of an enzyme that degrades chemical messengers causing smooth muscle relaxation. Two other drugs of this class will soon be available. This treatment was derived from basic consideration of smooth muscle physiology and trials of antihypertensive agents. The mechanism of action of this class of drugs has important implications for the entire vascular system.

Diabetes, erectile dysfunction, and failure of relaxation of smooth muscle appear to be interrelated. Impotent diabetics receiving intracavernous injection to induce erection may remain quite refractory with blood glucose levels over 300mg/dl. When glucose returns to normal levels, erectile ability returns in some cases—an important anecdotal observation. It seems that persistent smooth muscle contraction is present in hyperglycemia. Possibly, increased peripheral resistance promotes the peculiar diabetic distribution of atherosclerosis in arteries below the knee along with systemic hypertension commonly accompanying diabetes. High blood levels of glucose and insulin are growth factors for smooth muscle proliferation and at the same time promote vasoconstriction. Hypertension has been shown to relate to elevated insulin levels in type II diabetes. These hypotheses need further examination as they might suggest use of insulin-enhancing drugs rather than insulin itself. Adrenergic tone can be abolished by sympathetic ablation, an operation now in disuse but widely practiced in the past. I noted that sympathectomy done years before by my former chief, Dr. Holden, seemed to prevent later below-the-knee atherosclerosis on the index side, while the other non-sympathectomized side exhibited diffuse distal disease. This is certainly not an accident, for our study of disease processes shows that the distal disease is ordinarily quite symmetrically distributed. Given our virtual epidemic of diabetes, these are immensely promising observations and I would have wished to have an opportunity to investigate these aspects of diabetes more thoroughly.

VENOUS ULCERS: VEXING AND UNGLAMOROUS

Venous ulcers, long ago, were called "the opprobrium of the surgeon." Modern vascular surgeons have neglected venous disease. When Dr. John Davis left Western Reserve for Vermont, he left a group of patients with ulcers requiring tedious weekly dressing changes. I tried to do something about these patients flocking to my clinic. With the help of dedicated nurses, I developed operative approaches, which offered advances over Linton's classic procedure. These aimed to deflect or reduce elevated venous pressure in vulnerable areas, but without the need for extensive incisions that healed poorly. Along with improved conservative treatment, this approach led to healing of ulcers, and fewer patient visits. Dermatitis and ulcers in the lower leg near the ankle, so-called stasis changes, have several physiologic and anatomic causes. But these differences have not been recognized in evidence-based inquiries. In order to improve results, many cases require both ultrasound and contrast venous studies to select targets for surgical interventions. The efficacy of surgical versus conservative treatments, mainly compression and elevation, remains controversial, but when surgical intervention is possible, this, in my opinion, is a more effective way to treat patients. Surgical interventions, combined with optimal medical treatment, yielded long-term ulcer recurrences of about 10% in my experience compared to 15 to 50% for conservative treatment alone. Clinical nurse specialist Donna Kowallek and I used a crossover study to compare medical versus surgical intervention in a selected group of Reno patients. We demonstrated that ulcer recurrence and disability were greatly reduced in surgically treated patients.

While surgical innovations are based both on theory and empiric procedure changes, the integration of these two processes in the hands of skilled surgeons is no less elegant than the intricacies of cell biology. The process is also science of a high order. The science involved is finding out what interventions work in particular circumstances and discarding interventions that do not work in similar circumstances. In contrast to medication trials, prospective surgical trials are difficult to structure and harder to blind. Surgical technique is subtle; minor variations in approach by different operators can yield dramatically differing results.

We do know that transmission of venous hypertension to the skin and subcutis and white cell trapping promote "stasis changes" and skin ulceration. These processes can be controlled by a surgical approach in many instances. Medically, tetracycline derivatives and local steroids that inhibit inflammatory responses caused by white cell trapping offer another approach. One treatment should not preclude the other, but more work is needed to convince the medical community of favorable prospects for active treatment. Trials are needed to convince the medical community at large, and the statements about venous disease based on meta-analyses in current "evidence-based literature" almost border on the silly. Since blinded prospective studies have evolved as gold standard for "evidence-based medicine and surgery," the problem requires more work and a modicum of clinical intelligence. Vascular surgeons including Dr. Peter Glovitsky at the Mayo Clinic, Dr, John J. Bergan in San Diego, Drs. Robert Kisner and Bo Ecklôf in Hawaii, Dr. Jean Perrin and others in France, recognize this need. Unfortunately, granting agencies have yet to fund this research. Treatment of venous ulceration is a work in progress, which I hope to see completed.

UNFINISHED BUSINESS

Plastic grafts placed in the lower extremity fail more often than vein grafts. When a redo profunda artery to below-the-knee popliteal vein graft for limb salvage was done in 1983 and occluded three days postoperatively, the only alternative was replacing the main body of the failed vein graft with an expanded polytetrafluoroethylene (PTFE) graft. I left vein cuffs sutured to the arteries; this plastic graft remained patent for six years. About this time, Dr. Justin Miller of Adelaide, Australia, visited George Washington University to observe our approach to erectile dysfunction. It was then that I learned about his "Miller vein cuff." This variant and the "Taylor patch" appeared to prolong patency of PTFE grafts.

We examined the biology of vein-cuffed anastomoses in dog carotid arteries. Drs. William Suggs, Horace Henriques and I confirmed that vein cuffs enhanced graft patency and decreased myointimal hyperplasia at the sutured sites. Soon after, Dr. Anton Sidawy and I tested the hypothesis that the favorable effect might be due to minimizing compliance mismatch between the stiff graft and the artery. We encircled the vein cuff with another external PTFE cuff that limited expansion, thus recreating a compliance mismatch. The favorable effect of the vein cuff remained. We observed the effect of cuff geometry by creating a separate PTFE cuff to reproduce the geometry of a vein cuff; the altered geometry failed to yield a favorable result. We postulated that the vein cuff endothelium at the graft artery junction accounted for better patency. As my work progressed, I became more and more reluctant to sacrifice dogs, although I recognized that this was the only way to examine this kind of question. I could not begin to scrub until the animals were fully draped and out of view.

Mr. Peter L. Harris, a vascular consultant in England, showed theoretically favorable flow patterns in vitro with a funnel like configuration of a PTFE graft, much like that produced by a vein cuff. In England, it is difficult to obtain permission to work upon animals to test surgical hypotheses. These workers concluded that this configuration would offer better results and the grafts were marketed and widely sold. But human trials showed that the hooded plastic grafts were not particularly durable. For some reason, the endothelial lining is essential. Sidawy and Richard Neville in Washington simplified vein cuff construction in creating a balloon-like patch that demonstrated good intermediate results. While these evolutions of technique occurred in small steps, illustrating the science behind surgical innovations, no automatic method exists to find scientific truth for surgical applications. The process involves three steps: recognition of the problem, theories, and refutations. One undertaking remains—to discover how and why endothelial-lined cuffs offer favorable effects. Experimenting with vein cuffs devoid of endothelium might accomplish this.

I dismissed, overlooked and neglected concepts requiring reexamination. The idea about vasoconstriction in diabetic erectile dysfunction and its unique relationship to infracrural patterns of atherosclerosis needs work. Atherosclerotic plaque regression or stabilization with systemic treatment demands better definition. Energy metabolism in shock and endotoxemia requires reconsideration. The late Dr. Robert M. Zollinger purported that candidates for promotion to associate professor ought to have a number of peer-reviewed papers equal to their age. The publication of one minor observation sets the stage for more and more related minute annotations. Researchers are tempted to play variations on a theme, something that the late Dr. John Porter of Oregon called the "salami slicer" effect. Inciting deadlines and academic incentives are practical realities, but a major work with leading to unifying concepts, such as those accomplished by Darwin and Mendel, is clearly of more scientific value than numbers on a bibliography. I plead guilty to the numbers temptation, yet the many variations of disease seem to demand unique and specific approaches that cannot as yet be reduced to a unifying theory

Sometimes I see a fine tapestry in this past work; other times, I see a tattered rag. I become alternately pleased, then unhappy. Some quests, including the mitochondrial studies, were time-consuming and unrewarding interms of outcomes. I consider mitochondria as hummingbirds hover at a birdfeeder outside of my Virginia home. Long ago, I saw a picture, in the journal *Science,* of tightly packed mitochondria in the indefatigable hummingbird flight muscles that resembled the mitochondria in the muscle fibers of the mammalian diaphragm, a muscle that never tires. I think about these aerobic avian athletes and wonder what secrets they have to teach us about bioenergetics.

I am impatient with myself and with the delay in translating research to practice. In old files, I found a publication with the anesthesia group at Case Western Reserve University. We used systolic time intervals (STI) to measure the effects of anesthesia, aortic occlusion and unclamping on cardiac function. These were more effective in guiding intraoperative management than Swan Ganz catheters. We concluded: "The immediate detection and treatment of changes in left ventricular function add an important safety factor in minimizing cardiac mortality in aortic surgery." Carefully monitoring cardiac function, we performed one hundred consecutive aortic cases without a death. In spite of this observation, Swan Ganz catheters became routine rather than second-to-second monitoring of cardiac function. During this type of surgery, we require instantaneous monitoring. Swan Ganz catheters are mainly useful for longer-term fluid management. Only recently has ultrasound visualization of the left ventricular function been computerized and routinely employed to monitor cardiac performance.

Past randomized trials have presented the public and the profession with perplexing data, but trial performances and interpretations are improving. Trial data cannot unerringly guide doctors dealing with individuals in their examining rooms. Although level 1 evidence has yielded some remarkable epidmiologic insights, I worry about some of the results, which are not in accord with experimental evidence. For example, antioxidant supplementation with ascorbic acid and vitamin E, overall, has not been found to have an effect on coronary death, but these agents actually regulate cytokine production by macrophages and reduce so-called oxidative stress. Work by Dr. Byron McGregor in Reno, showing dramatic cytokine responses to cells exposed to vitamins C and E, resides in abstract form. I became a convert to vitamin C use after an airplane trip from San Francisco to New York while sitting next to Dr. Linus Pauling. He asked what we did about vitamin supplementation after surgery. I told him we gave six to ten times the usual daily doses of the water-soluble vitamins with our intravenous fluids. Beaming, he said that I was the first doctor that he had met who did this, then, he asked why. I replied, "Because my boss, Dr. Holden, told me to." A stack of reprints about vitamin C ten inches thick sits in my bookcase, and I do not know what to advise. Some suggest that excess vitamin C might be harmful; like aspirin, we still do not know the proper dose of vitamin C.

A prospective randomized Veterans Administration study, "The Iron and Atherosclerosis Study (FeAST)," chaired by Dr. Leo Zacharski, is now testing the effect of reduction of iron stores in stable claudicants using measured bleeding. Men, and postmenopausal women, accumulate excess iron stores. Iron in ferrous form is a powerful oxidizing and inflammatory agent that possibly contributes an inflammatory stimulus to atherogenesis. Dr. Jerome L. Sullivan, in 1981, cited evidence that accumulation of excess iron appeared to relate to coronary disease in men and to postmenopausal women. The Veterans Administration initiated FeAST in 1999 to test this hypothesis. The aim is to see if phlebotomy will affect the course of atherosclerosis, including death from heart attack and stroke in stable but symptomatic individuals.

We at the VA in Reno received permission to measure serum cytokines TNF-alpha, its receptors and interleukins 2, 6 and 10 in FeAST subjects and to compare these to healthy controls. We would also be able to determine whether phlebotomy might affect this pattern. A vascular nurse practitioner, Virginia W. Hayes, energized this work. We uncovered an inflammatory cytokine signature in our atherosclerotics and found that reducing iron stores appeared to lower elevated inflammatory cytokine levels. We continue to observe the clinical outcomes.

It will be astonishing to discover that bleeding, a relic of medicine's dark ages, could offer a beneficial effect on inflammation and irritation promoting atherosclerosis. In view of our work on lipids, confirmation of markers of inflammation in atherosclerosis helps us understand what might be the final parts of the puzzle.

I remain ambivalent about past work; the life of the mind has given me some of my best and my worst hours. I agonize over why I did not go further with this or that project. I question whether my work made any difference at all. The same original ideas appeared simultaneously to others and progress would have occurred in any event. In darker moments, I muse that surgeons might best concentrate on flawless technical performances. As Yogi Bera said, "You can't hit and think." Intellectual pretensions offer an escape hatch for an inadequate surgeon and a distraction for a competent one. The life of the mind in the surgical setting is perhaps too stimulating, and, surgeons used to making decisions based on incomplete evidence, risk acceptance of potentially bad science. Much is at stake in the operative act—sutures placed sloppily or tied too tightly, or a moment's distraction, can compromise life or limb. Discipline is needed, yet discipline must not be so harsh as to stifle the creative spirit. There must also be generosity in supporting novel ideas, a trait most surgeons display.

Clinicians who probe basic science issues require technically competent scientific collaborators and the clinicians themselves must be competent scientists. Employment of "captive" departmental Ph.D. grant-writers may be practical, but not optimal. Clearly, a host of talented Ph.D. investigators contribute richly to biological science; some would say that their contributions, focused and disciplined as they are, might even be better science. However, solutions for clinical problems might more readily come from those who intimately understand disease processes and have a sense of urgency in seeking solutions. A Ph.D. prominence on grant review panels, while adding rigor, can exert a stifling effect on clinical research and also says something about the scientific motivations of a new generation of clinicians. The search for collaboration must be completely voluntary. Personal taste, inspiration, and circumstance, much like love, all influence the choice of a research problem. Each or all can be valid motives. However, a problem may be chosen, the opportunity to pursue a life of the mind is an extraordinary privilege. And when a clinician chooses this path, something good may actually come of it.

REFERENCES

DePalma RG, DePalma MT and DeForest M. Experimental alteration of the shape of rabbit ear cartilage. J Surg Res 1964; 4:2-6

DePalma RG, Reid WM and Fitzpatrick HF. The relation of d-pantothenyl alcohol therapy to the resumption of intestinal function postoperatively. Am J Surg 1964; 107:813-815.

Gallstones and Biliary Dynamics

DePalma RG and Hubay CA. A Comparative study of the surface activity of human and canine bile. Surg Gynecol Obstet 1964; 118:1248-1252

DePalma RG and Levey S: Arborization patterns in human bile. Nature 207 1965; 637-638

DePalma R, Hubay CA and Levey S: The micellar properties of bile. JAMA 1966; 195: 943-945

DePalma RG, Hubay CA and Insull W Jr. The effect of T tube drainage of cholesterol and bile acid metabolism in man. Surg Gynecol Obstet 123:269-273, 1966

DePalma RG, Levey S, Hartman P and Hubay CA. Bile acids and serum cholesterol following T tube drainage. Arch Surg 1967; 94:271-276

Cussler EL, Evans D, Fennell A, and DePalma RG. A model for gall bladder function and cholesterol gallstone formation. Proc Nat'l Acad Sci 1970; 67:400-407

Evans DF, DePalma RG, Nadas J and Thomas J. The conductance of bile salt-lecithin-water mixtures. J Sol Chem 1972; 1:377-386

Atherosclerosis

DePalma RG, Hubay CA, Vogt C, Insull W Jr, Hartman P, and Robinson AV. Regression and prevention of experimental atherosclerosis: Effects of diet and bile diversion in the dog. Surg Forum 1968; 19:308-310

DePalma RG, Hubay CA, Robinson AV and Hartman PH. Regression of hypercholesterolemia and atherosclerosis: Biliary diversion and dietary changes in the dog. Surg Forum 1969; 20:392-393

DePalma RG, Hubay CA, Insull W Jr, Robinson AV and Hartman PH. Progression and regression of experimental atherosclerosis. Surg Gynecol Obstet 1970; 131:633-547

DePalma RG, Hubay CA, Botti RE and Peterka JL. Treatment of surgical patients with atherosclerosis and hyperlipdemia. Surg Gynecol Obstet; 1970: 131:313-322

Wray R, DePalma RG and Hubay CA: Late occlusion of aortofemoral bypass grafts: Influence of cigarette smoking. Surgery 1971; 70:969-973

DePalma RG, Insull W Jr, Bellon EM, Roth WT and Robinson AV. Animal models for study of progression and regression of atherosclerosis. Surgery 1972; 72:268-278

DePalma RG, Bellon EM, Insull W Jr, Roth WT and Robinson AV. Studies on progression and regression of experimental atherosclerosis: Techniques and application to the rhesus monkey. Med Primatology (Karger Basel) III 1972; 313-323

Rosen AB, DePalma RG and Victor Y: Risk factors in peripheral atherosclerosis. Arch Surg 1973; 107: 303-307

DePalma RG, Bellon EM, Klein L, Koletsky S and Insull W Jr. Approaches to evaluating regression of experimental atherosclerosis. In Manning GM and Haust MD (Eds): Atherosclerosis: Metabolic, Morphologic and Clinical Aspects. New York, Plenum Publishing 1977; pp 459-470

DePalma RG, Koletsky S, Bellon EM, and Insull W Jr. Failure of regression of atherosclerosis in dogs with moderate cholesterolemia. Atherosclerosis 27 1977; 297-310

DePalma RG and Clowes AW: Interventions in atherosclerosis: A review for surgeons. Surgery 1978; 175-189

DePalma RG, Bellon EM, Koletsky S and Schneider DL. Atherosclerotic plaque regression in rhesus monkeys induced by bile acid sequestrant. Exp Molec Pathol 1979; 31:423-439

DePalma RG, Klein L, Bellon EM and Koletsky S. Regression of atherosclerotic plaques in rhesus monkeys. Arch Surg 1980; 115:1268-1278

Bomberger RA, DePalma RG and Ambrose TA. Aspirin and dipyridamol inhibit endothelial healing. Arch Surg 1982; 117 1459-1464

Bomberger RA, Wilburn J and DePalma RG. Aspirin and dipyridamole increase intimal thickening after injury. Surg Forum 34 1983; 475-477

DePalma RG, Bellon EM, Manalo P, and Bomberger RA. Failure of antiplatelet treatment in dietary atherosclerosis: A serial intervention study. In Gallo LL and Vahouny GV (Eds): Cardiovascular Disease: Molecular and Cellular Mechanisms, Prevention, Treatment. New York, Plenum Press1987; pp 407-426

Shock

Holden WD, DePalma RG, Drucker WR and McKalen A. Ultrastructural changes in hemorrhagic shock. Ann Surg 1965; 162: 517-536

DePalma RG, Coil J, Davis JH and Holden WD. Cellular and ultrastructural changes in endotoxemia: A light and electron microscopic study. Surgery 1967; 62:505-515

DePalma RG, Drucker WR, Levey S, Polster DR and Holden WD. Histochemical investigation of hepatic adenosinetriphosphatase and glucose-6-phosphatase activity in hemorrhagic shock. Proc Soc Exp Biol Med 1968; 127:1090-1094

Harano Y, DePalma RG and Miller M. Fatty acid oxidation, citric acid cycle activity, and morphology of mitochondria in diabetic rat liver. Proc Soc Exp Biol Med 1969; 131:913-917

DePalma RG, Levey S and Holden WD. Ultrastructural and oxidative phosphorylation of liver mitochondria in experimental hemorrhagic shock. J Trauma 1970; 10:122-234

DePalma RG, Robinson AV and Holden WD: Fluid therapy in hemorrhagic shock: Experimental evaluation. J Surg Oncol 1970; 2:349-357

DePalma RG, Harano Y, Robinson AV and Holden WD: Structure and function of hepatic mitochondria in hemorrhage and endotoxemia. Surg Forum 1970; 21:3-5

DePalma RG, Holden WD and Robinson AV: Fluid therapy in experiment hemorrhagic shock: Ultrastructural effects in liver and muscle. Ann Surg 1972; 175:539-551

Harano Y, DePalma RG, Lavine L and Miller M: Fatty acid oxidation, oxidative phosphorylation and ultrastructure of mitochondria in the diabetic rat liver: Hepatic factors in diabetic ketosis. Diabetes 1972; 21:257-270

Rhodes RS, DePalma RG and Robinson AV. Intestinal barrier function in hemorrhagic shock. J Surg Res 1973; 14:305-312

Rhodes RS, DePalma RG, and Robinson AV. The relationship of critical uptake volume to energy production and endotoxemia in late hemorrhagic shock. Am J Surg 1975; 130:560-564

Rhodes S and DePalma RG. Reversal of ischemically induced uncoupled oxidative phosphorylation by restoration of adequate perfusion. Surg Forum 27:13-15, 1976

DePalma RG, Glickman MH, Hartman P and Robinson AV: Prevention of endotoxin induced changes in oxidative phosphorylation in hepatic mitochondria. Surgery 1977; 82:68-73

Rhodes RS, DePalma RG and Druet RL: Reversibility of ischemically induced mitochondrial dysfunction with perfusion. Surg Gynecol Obstet 1977; 145:719-724

Hoffman M, Avellone JC, Plecha FR, Rhodes RS, Donovan DL, Beven EG, DePalma RG and Frisch JA: Operation for ruptured abdominal aortic aneurysms: A community-wide experience. Surgery 1982; 91:597-602

Bomberger RA, McGregor B and DePalma RG: Optimal fluid replacement after aortic reconstruction: A prospective study. J Vasc Surg 4:164-167, 1986

Erectile Dysfunction

DePalma RG, Levine SB, and Feldman S. Preservation of erectile function after aortoiliac reconstruction. Arch Surg 1978; 113:958-962

DePalma RG, Kedia K and Persky L. Vascular operations for preservation of sexual function. In Bergan JJ and Yao JST (Eds): The Surgery of the Aorta and Its Body Branches. New York, Grune and Stratton, Inc. 1979 pp 227-296

DePalma RG, Kedia K and Persky L: Surgical options in the correction of vasculogenic impotence. Vasc Surg 1980; 14:92-103

DePalma RG and Merchant RF. Vascular operations and preservation of sexual function. In Greenhalgh RM (ed): Proceedings of International Symposium on Hormones and Vascular Disease. London, England, Pitman Publishers1981; pp 306-218

Merchant RF Jr and DePalma RG. The effects of femoro-femoral grafts on postoperative sexual function. Correlation with penile pulse volume recordings. Surgery 1981; 90:962-970

DePalma RG: Impotence in vascular disease: Relationship to vascular surgery. Brit J Surg 1982; 69:514-516

DePalma RG: Etiology and management of sexual problems related to aorto-iliac disease and surgery. In Veith FJ (ed): Critical Problems in Vascular Surgery. New York, Appleton Century Crofts 1982; pp 429-443

Stauffer D and DePalma RG: A comparison of penile-brachial index (PBI) and penile pulse volume recordings (PVR) for diagnosis of vasculogenic impotence. Bruit 1983; 7:29-32

DePalma RG: Preserving erectile function after aorto-iliac surgery: State of the art. Contem Surg 1983; 23:65-68

DePalma RG: Arterial reconstructive procedures for impotence. Rev Brasil de Angiol e Cir Vasc 1986; 16:83-86

DePalma RG and Edwards C: Screening for pelvic arterial disease. In Balas P (ed): Progress in Angiology. Milan, Italy, Edizioni Minerva Medica 1986; pp 483-485

DePalma RG and Edwards C: Noninvasive evaluation of erectile dysfunction and intracorporal papaverine injection. In Virag R and Virag H (Eds): Proceedings of First World Conference on Impotence. Paris, France, Editions du CERI 1986; pp 115-119

DePalma RG, Emsellem HA, Edwards CM, Druy EM, Shultz SW, Miller HC and Bergsrud D: A screening sequence for vasculogenic impotence. J Vasc Surg 1987; 5:228-236

DePalma RG, Schwab F, Druy EM, Miller HC and Emsellem HA: Experience in diagnosis and treatment of impotence caused by cavernosal leak syndrome. J Vasc Surg 1989, 10:117-121

DePalma RG, Schwab FJ, Emsellem HA, Massarin E, and Bergsrud D: Noninvasive assessment of impotence. In Pearce WH and Yao JST (Eds): The Surgical Clinics of North America. Philadelphia, W.B. Saunders Company, VV/70 1990; pp 119-131

DePalma RG, Schwab FJ, Emsellem HA, Massarin E, Bergsrud D, Olding M: Vascular Interventions for Impotence: Effect of a Screening Sequence. Int J Impot Research 1990: 2:358-359

Yu GW, Schwab FJ, Melograna F, Miller HC, DePalma RG: Pre and Post-Operative Dynamic Cavernosography: Objective assessment of venous ligation for impotence. Int J Impot Research 1990; 1:379-380

DePalma RG, Michal V: Point of View: Deja Vu—Again: Advantages and Limitations of Methods for Assessing Penile Arterial Flow. Urology 1990; 36:199-200

DePalma RG, Gomez CA, Dalton C, Schwab FJ, Miller HC: Predictive Value of a Screening Sequence for Venous Impotence. In Austoni E, Wagner G (Eds) Int J of Impot Res 1992; London, Smith-Gordon and Company, Ltd, pp 122-123

Yu GW, Schwab FJ, Melograna FS, DePalma RG, Miller HC, Rickholt AL. Preoperative and Postoperative Dynamic Cavernosography and Cavernosometry: objective assessment of venous ligation for impotence. Journal of Urology 1992, 147:618-622

DePalma RG: Impotence: Invited commentary on NIH consensus conference. Int J Impot Res 1994; 5:222-224

DePalma RG and Olding MJ: Surgery for Vasculogenic Impotence in *Vascular and Endovascular Surgical Techniques* 3rd Edition. Greenhalgh RM (ed) London WB Saunders 1994; 239-244

DePalma RG: The role of the vascular surgeon in diagnosis and treatment of impotence. Eur J Vasc Endovasc Surg; 1995, 9:4-6

DePalma RG, Olding M, Yu GW, Schwab FJ, Druy EM, Miller HC, Massarin EH: Vascular Interventions for Impotence: Lessons Learned. J Vascular Surgery, 1995; 21:576-585

DePalma RG: New Developments in the diagnosis and treatment of impotence. West J Med 1996; 164:54-61

DePalma RG: Editorial Comment: Has the efficacy of penile arterial by-pass surgery in the treatment of arteriogenic erectile dysfunction been determined? Int J Impot Res 1996; 8:251-252

DePalma RG: Vascular Surgery for impotence: a review. Int J of Impot Res 1997; 9:61-67

DePalma RG: Expert opinion: The best treatment for impotence. Vasc Surgery 1998, 32:519-521

DePalma RG: Iliac Artery Occlusive Disease: Impotence and Colon Ischemia in *Endovascular Surgery, Third Edition* Ed Moore WS, Ahn SS, Philadelphia, WB Saunders Co 2001: pp355-360

Venous Ulcer: A vexing problem

DePalma RG: Surgical therapy for venous stasis. Surgery 1974; 76:910-917

DePalma RG: Surgical therapy for venous stasis: Results of a modified Linton operation. Am J Surg 1979; 137:810-813

DePalma RG: Surgical Treatment of Chronic Venous Ulceration. In Bergan JJ and Yao JST (Eds): Venous Disorders, Philadelphia, W.B. Saunders Company 1990; pp 396-406

DePalma RG: Surgical Treatment of Chronic Venous Ulceration. In Martimbeau-Raymond P, Prescott R, Zummo M (Eds): Phlebology 92, Volume 2. London, John Libbey and Company, Ltd 1992; pp 1235-1237

DePalma RG: Evolving Surgical Approaches for Venous Ulceration. In Negus D, Jantet G, Coleridge-Smith PD (Eds) Phlebology 95, Berlin, Springer-Verlag. Phlebologie, 1995; Suppl. I: 980-982

DePalma RG: Kowallek DL: Venous Ulceration: A cross over study from non-operative to operative treatment. J Vasc Surg 1996; 24:788-79

DePalma RG: Do primary varicose veins lead to ulceration? Vascular Surgery 1996; 30:1-3

DePalma RG: Management of incompetent perforators: conventional techniques in *Handbook of Venous Disorders* Ed Gloviczki P, Yao JST. London. Chapman and Hall 1996; pp 471-480

Kowallek DL, DePalma RG: Venous ulceration: active approaches to treatment. J Vasc Nurs 1997; 15:50-57

DePalma RG: Linton's operation and the modification of open techniques in : *Atlas of Endoscopic Vein Surgery* Eds Glovitsky P and Bergan JJ. New York. Springer, 1997; pp 107-116

Kowallek DL, DePalma RG: A new approach to an old problem: Subfascial Endoscopic Perforator Surgery. J Vasc Nursing 1999; 17:65-70

DePalma RG: Trophic disorders and venous leg ulcer in Chronic Venous Insufficiency. Phlebolymphology 1999; 22: pp 2-3

DePalma RG, Kowallek DL, Barcia TC, Cafferata HT: Target selection for surgical treatment of severe chronic venous insufficiency: Comparison of duplex scanning and phlebography. J Vas Surg 2000; 32:913-20

DePalma RG, Kowallek DL, Barcia TC: New approaches to an old and vexing problem: Improving the results of SEPS: An Overview. Acta chir belg 2000; 100:100-103

Unfinished Business

Suggs WD, Henriques HF and DePalma RG. Vein cuff interposition prevents juxta-anastomotic neointimal hyperplasia. Ann Surg 1988; 207:717-723

Sidawy AN, Norberto JI, DePalma RG, Trad KS, Neville RS, Najjar S, Jones BA. The protective effect of vein-cuffed anastomoses is not mechanical in origin. J Vasc Surg 1995; 21:558-565

DePalma RG, Talieh YJ: Infrainguinal reconstruction in Diabetes. Diabetes 1996; 45 (Suppl 3) S126-S128

Dauchot PJ, DePalma RG, Geum D and Canella J. Detection and prevention of cardiac dysfunction during aortic surgery. J Surg Res 1979; 26:574-580

The Iron and Atherosclerosis Trial

Sullivan JL. Iron and the sex difference in heart disease risk. Lancet 1981; 1:1293-1294

Howes PS, Zacharski LR, Sullivan J and Chow B. Role of stored iron in atherosclerosis. J Vasc Nurs 2000; 18:109-116

DePalma RG, Hayes VW, Cafferata HT, Mohammadpour BS, Chow BK, Zacharski LR, Hall MR. Cytokine signatures in atherosclerotic claudicants. J Surg Res 2003; 111: 215-21

CARING FOR THE GREATEST GENERATION

This generation of Americans has a rendezvous
with destiny.
Franklin Delano Roosevelt, cited by Brokaw

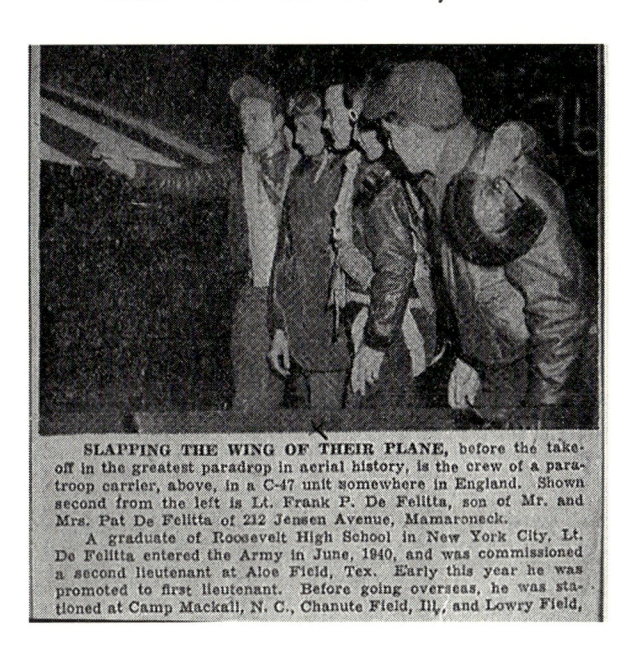

> **SLAPPING THE WING OF THEIR PLANE**, before the take-off in the greatest paradrop in aerial history, is the crew of a paratroop carrier, above, in a C-47 unit somewhere in England. Shown second from the left is Lt. Frank P. De Felitta, son of Mr. and Mrs. Pat De Felitta of 212 Jensen Avenue, Mamaroneck.
> A graduate of Roosevelt High School in New York City, Lt. De Felitta entered the Army in June, 1940, and was commissioned a second lieutenant at Aloe Field, Tex. Early this year he was promoted to first lieutenant. Before going overseas, he was stationed at Camp Mackall, N. C., Chanute Field, Ill., and Lowry Field,

The Herald Statesman, Yonkers, New York, May 1944

Long before they came to be known as the "greatest generation," they were simply our older brothers, cousins and uncles. We, neighborhood kids, sitting on my stoop in August 1945, heard that a large bomb had been dropped in Japan. I remember the exact moment that an excited older boy ran across Kimball Avenue to give us that news. After a second bomb was dropped, the entire nation seemed to sigh with relief. Japan surrendered: the war was over. The men who had returned from Europe did not have to go to the Pacific to face a fanatical enemy in a bloody island war. They all came back to the Bronx and Yonkers wearing medals. My cousin Frankie DeFelitta, who flew C-47 transports for the invasion of Europe, returned wearing a glamorous squashed aviator's cap and a Distinguished Flying Cross. Another serviceman, Joe Pontronio, came back in a tight-fitting infantryman's uniform and shiny combat boots wearing a Congressional Medal of Honor. He looked wild-eyed, and you would not want to meet him in a dark alley. He had killed scores of Germans in a machine gun nest. They were heroes, and we admired them. We were only twelve or thirteen years old when they came back to our adolescent worship. We did not know then that Mr. Brokaw would call them the "greatest generation" but we knew that they were great men. We were all sorry that we too had not had the chance to fight.

Cousin Frankie let me hang out with him and I was so proud to be with him. We hung around Fordham Road in the Bronx, went to Lowe's Paradise, to Poe Park, and visited friends in the old neighborhood. When I was thirteen, Frankie taught me to drive an old 1935 Buick that he had resurrected in Mamaroneck, New York. With true pilot's care, he let me drive solo in an empty lot near our house in Yonkers. We tried to emulate these heroes, so we all started smoking. Everyone in those days smoked, it was just an adult thing to do, and it was also "cool." We mimicked the styles of Humphrey Bogart, James Cagney and Edward G. Robinson, as we dragged deeply on Lucky Strikes, Camels or long Pall Malls. We were becoming addicted, but we didn't know this then. Only after I became a physician caring for World War II veterans suffering from lung cancer, emphysema and vascular disease, did I grasp the dangers of this habit. After a rotation at the Veterans Hospital in Cleveland, I quit smoking at age thirty-three.

Cousin Frankie remained a cautious hero. Every pilot in his squadron, except him and one other man in it, had been shot down. Once I got him to take me to Playland in Rye, New York.

The war had left its mark on him. We went for a roller coaster ride and just as the cars started to roll, Frankie called out to the operator to stop the cars. Since it was a weekday, we were all alone on the train. He turned to the man controlling the ride with a large lever and asked, "Has anyone ever been killed on this thing?" The man replied, "Not for twenty years." The attendant was about to release the lever again when Cousin Frank asked, "What happened twenty years ago?" The attendant replied, "The park wasn't here." We went on our roller coaster ride, but I knew that Frankie had faced death and was still thinking about it.

When I came back to Reno in 1994, rather than doing private practice in town, I decided to devote all my efforts as full time chief of surgery at our Veterans Administration Hospital. We needed to get surgery back on track. The little white hospital nestled in the valley was then a visible and picturesque landmark but, except for intensive care, the operating room suite, and radiology, the bed facility was old. Its four bed wards, hot in the summer and drafty in the winter, were flanked by a few common bathrooms. A new building had been promised for years. Finally, under the direction of Mr. Gary Whitfield, an energetic and spirited man, and Mr.John Hempel, the associate director, much time was devoted to making this promise come true. I was impressed with these administrators, in contrast to those I had known in the private sector, who mainly worried about the size of their next bonus. The VA administrators were not motivated by money and spared no effort in learning everything they could about the needs of sick veterans. Gary spent a lot of time in airplanes, going to Washington, D.C., to lobby for the new building. New construction was difficult for the agency in 1994 and 1995. In spite of seven or eight years of promises, Reno might not get an updated hospital. New construction was discouraged nationally because the "greatest generation," now in their seventh and eighth decades of life, was dying off. In the Washoe Valley, however, our veteran population was growing, as was the case volume we saw. Against the odds, the new bed tower was completed in 1998.

Our efforts almost ended when Senator Allen Simpson from Wyoming visited Reno. In a nay-saying, penny-pinching way, he did not see why Northern Nevada veterans needed a new hospital. Simpson had also managed to close down Wyoming's medical school. I met with Simpson's staffers, along with Dr. Kenneth Madsen, a fourth-year resident and the son of a prominent attorney in Wyoming, and Dr. H. Treat Cafferata, the son-in-law of Barbara Vucanovich, a Republican congresswoman. We pointed out that, in Wyoming, there was no facility to train a promising young man like Ken Madsen. Neither did we have the facility to take proper care of our growing veteran population in Northern Nevada. The building finally went up. The hospital now became a modern facility, no longer an old-fashioned white elephant but a beautiful amber tan, a distinctly Western color. Joe Dobson, in maintenance, planted beautiful gardens about the area with minimal expense.

Veterans flocked to our new clinic and hospital building. They had always been loyal to this hospital even when it provided poor in-patient accommodations. A caring and hardworking nursing staff probably contributed to this loyalty. In contrast to the Washington experience, where secretaries squabbled and placed phones on an answering service, Doris Eyheralde, our surgical service secretary, tended our telephones promptly and cheerfully. Mr. Donald Barr, an amiable former marine, provided administrative support and taught me how to use the computer system. Dr. Todd Arcomano, recruited from Washington, D.C., cared for veterans in an exemplary manner. Todd, a fine surgeon and an honor graduate of Georgetown University, was the kind of doctor who always made patients feel good no matter how grave the illness. I had worked with him at the Veterans Hospital in Washington, D.C.. He was the kind of young man that every father would like to have for a son.

We had troubles with finances; all hospitals did for these were difficult times. One instance occurred just as I arrived from Washington in 1994. For reasons of budget, we were not able to hire the new academic general surgeon we had planned upon. The second serious crisis happened during budget year 1997-1998. In contrast to the obscure and confused way the financial problems were handled at George Washington, the financial details were played out by administration with all the cards on the table. The flow of funds in a large agency such as the VA is not always uniform and, further, is subject to congressional oversight. The shutting down of government agencies during that time was disruptive, but during these crises, all options were explored openly and rationally, and with final good results. Our third faculty member was hired.

Another aspect of a sound institution is the handling of personnel problems when an individual has an illness or bad luck. I had been ill for months with right flank pain, fevers, and urinary urgency thought to be due to a prostate infection. In early 1998, my wife, Eve, came out to take care of me during what I thought was simply a bad case of flu. This illness turned out to be an appendix that had ruptured in the pelvis, impinging upon my bladder. Dr. Arcomano and Dr. Lindsay Smith operated on me at Washoe Medical Center and did a great job in getting me through that surgical crisis, but I had to take a great deal of kidding. I really never had any symptoms of appendicitis until a mass appeared in my lower right abdomen. Some of my less gentle colleagues suggested I reread Cope's *Diagnosis of the Acute Abdomen*. At one point, I awoke from a delirium to find my friend, Father Frank Hoffmann, the pastor of Our Lady of Wisdom, praying over me. I decided that it was time to go to confession and a little later, I did just that. All during this time, I had the support of my friends at the hospital, and, during a prolonged recovery, I was able to continue work, completing two book chapters and initiating the proposal that led us to get a cooperative study grant.

Six years in Reno, from 1994 to the fall of 2000, passed in the blink of an eye. The Biggest Little City still was much as I had left it in 1982, except that the town had grown considerably and seemed more sophisticated. I listened to 1950s music on my car radio as I drove down to the hospital from the foothills. I cherished my little time warp and felt young again. I renewed old friendships with the surgeons in town and Dr. Pacita Manalo, a fine pathologist who had contributed to our research on atherosclerosis in monkeys. I made new friends, too. Treat, Gary, and I attended Rotary Club downtown at Harrah's for weekly luncheon meetings. Rotary might seem corny to some sophisticates, but this service club was great. Its members' efforts were simple and heartfelt, and they were sincere in trying to serve the community, as well as taking on international challenges. As we did old-fashioned American things, I felt the way I did when I was a boy in school. It felt good to stand up, say a prayer, pledge to the American flag and sing "God Bless America." The downtown Rotary in Reno did an enormous amount for the community. I met the mayor, the former mayor, the sheriff, the district attorney, and other luminaries. I got more from Rotary than I ever gave. I wished that I could have been of more service, but the surgical schedule was busy. I paid dues and fines conscientiously and showed up for lunch when I could.

During this time, I was often reluctant to leave town for professional obligations because something was always going on at home. The National Championship Air Races at Stead followed hot August nights, a parade of antique automobiles that I had grown up with. I fell in love with a 1933 Plymouth Coupe, but resisted the temptation to relive my high school years. Then, there were the hot air balloon races. It was a beautiful thing to wake up early and to see the balloons ascending in the dawn patrol with the Sierra as a backdrop. It was even more fun to go up in a balloon, an eerie experience as compared to flying an airplane, and we were never sure where we would land. We went boating and swimming in Lake Tahoe, shot skeet and sporting clays in the mountains and went on cross-country four-wheel drives in the mountains and in the deserts. The opera and the chamber orchestra performances began in the fall. Saturdays and Sundays, the weekend movie club met, including the Brighams, Edna and Robert, as well as Frankie Sue Del Papa, our attorney general. Since these were very persuasive women, Bob Brigham and I saw lots of "chick flicks," but we also saw most of the academy award winners. I finally got elected to the Prospectors' Club. My name had been on the list for fifteen years. It was harder to get into the Prospectors' than it was to be admitted to the Cosmos Club of Washington. I was elected with the support of Dr. Ernest Mack, member number 1, and Dr. H. Treat Cafferata.

The busy surgical schedule at the Veterans Hospital grew to about one thousand cases a year. A fine group of residents, recruited to the University of Nevada training program, benefited educationally. These young doctors spent an average of sixteen months during five years at the VA Hospital in Reno. Two of my favorites became vascular surgeons. Initially, some of the young doctors lived with me at 2001 Lakeridge. Later, the hospital secured fine accommodations for them at a nearby motel. New faculty members joined us—Patricia Eubanks-May and Treat Cafferata came to teach full time, and Dr. Michael Gainey provided general thoracic backup. The resident deployment was later to change in favor of Southern Nevada and this ultimately affected my personal decision-making.

We were academically productive in the area of vascular disease. Our work in venous disease was well received nationally and internationally. Assisted by Donna Stauffer Kowallek, a vascular nurse, we demonstrated the efficacy of perforator interruption along with correction of deep insufficiency for treatment of venous ulceration, a vexing and troublesome problem. We published three papers in the *Journal of Vascular Surgery*. Donna's meticulous care of these difficult patients allowed us to report a crossover study comparing surgical with medical treatment. I believe the approach will stand the test of time. Tragically, Donna became ill in 1998, developing a severe headache and quickly succumbing to a glioblastoma. We all mourned her.

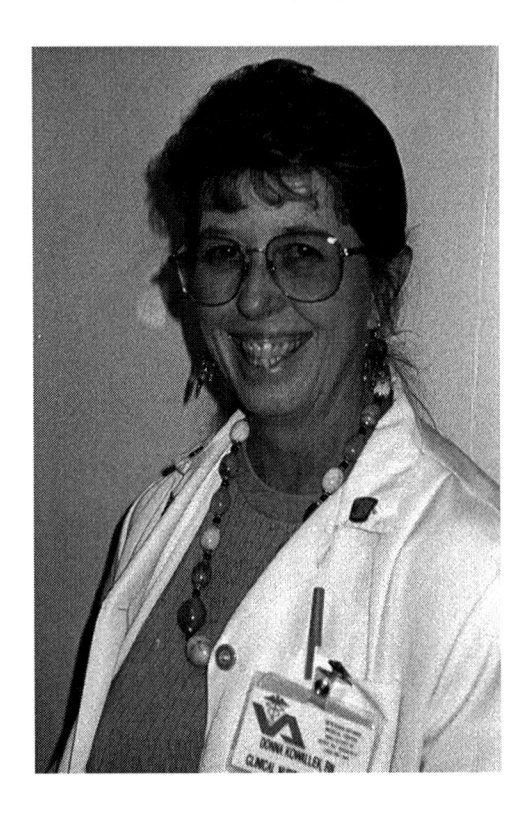

Donna Stauffer Kowallek, RN

We joined an exciting new VA Cooperative Study, FeAST, to test the hypothesis that excess iron stores might be a risk factor in progressive atherosclerosis. It was thought that measured bleeding might relieve this progression. A newly qualified vascular nurse practitioner, Ms. Virginia Hayes, fiercely dedicated to the care of veterans, spearheaded the study, making it possible. She helped Donna in her last days and now carries on a fine nursing tradition in the care of patients suffering from vascular disease. Atherosclerosis and cancer are the two nemeses of the "greatest generation." We recognized that the best treatment for patients with vascular disease below the inguinal ligament was exercise, cessation of smoking, and optimal medical treatment. We began to randomize patients to see relief of excess iron stores made a difference in disease progression. Clearly, there was something more beyond elevated cholesterol in these patients with advanced disease. As part of this, we began a search for proinflammatory cytokines among this group of patients who will be followed for years to come. A clear proinflammatory pattern emerged in the group of Nevada veterans with vascular disease.

During this time, the Veterans Health Administration changed radically and we were on the forefront of this change. Veterans hospitals were no longer domiciliary facilities with leisurely patient turnovers. The agency took a hard look at ways to provide better health care services. Prodded by performance standards, our average hospital length of stay declined to an average of about four and a half days. We did many of our operations as outpatient procedures and certain types of major surgical cases were admitted directly to the operating room. Attention to new performance standards made us take a hard look at our work and, I believe, made us as good or better than the private sector. From 1998 to 2000, we made a transition, albeit painful, to computerized medical records, greatly facilitating tracking and follow-up of patients. The agency was decentralized into VISNs (Veterans Integrated Service Networks) and as a member of VISN 21, the Sierra Nevada Health Care Network, we gauged our performance against other hospitals in our VISN and the other twenty-two VISNs within the country.

Beginning in 1993, surgical outcomes were methodically tracked using NSQIP (National Surgical Quality Improvement Program) that calculated mortality and morbidity on a risk-adjusted basis. This made for an even playing field, taking into account comorbidities. Initially, some surgeons resisted this close scrutiny of surgical results. Having had experience with the Cleveland Vascular Registry, I welcomed these outcome analyses, and later, most surgical services looked forward to receiving these data, which led to improved processes and structure of care. As one of my Cleveland colleagues put it, "Outcome is everything." The goal of surgery must be to get the patient out of the hospital intact and alive, and not in a box. However, some old surgical platitudes have to disappear. Among the worst are, "If no one is dying, you are not operating," or, "These things happen," or, "We really didn't want to operate, but the patient (the family) wanted it."

NSQIP is the first nationally organized risk adjusted quality assurance program permitting objective comparisons of surgical outcomes. Services in our system experiencing problems could be identified and corrected. Our mortality in Reno was low, though morbidity would vary depending on how many high-risk patients required surgical treatment. Good results are more than a matter of surgical skill and careful preoperative preparation. Surgical results also depend upon a fine intensive care unit staff, medical consultants, and anesthesiologists. A remarkably skilled anesthesia department headed by Dr. Joseph Bovill, including Drs. Colin Tredrea, Agi Melton, and my friend from the old days, Massoud Dorostkar, helped us operate successfully upon high risk and critically ill individuals.

Seven years at the Reno VA seemed to fly by. The "greatest generation" continued to be a pleasure to care for. We heard that they were dying at the rate of 1,000 daily throughout the United States. They remained as brave as they were in World War II and as intrepid in facing the infirmities of death and old age as they had been in facing the perils of the battlefield. Compared to private patient experience, these men were a privilege to care for. Others followed them. Korean veterans were very similar to the World War II veterans, perhaps a bit more reticent. Vietnam veterans did not really trust the government, so Veterans Hospitals were only attracting 10 to 15% of them. We tried even harder with this group. While I was taking a detailed history from a Vietnam veteran, he said with tears in his eyes, "You really seem to care about us." These veterans had unique burdens of post-traumatic stress disorder, cigarette addiction, and were affected by the drug culture of that conflict and that time. They were not welcomed home as were the World War veterans. Many in the Reno area were homeless, having dropped out of society altogether.

I had envisioned staying in Reno, this beautiful little town tucked against the eastern slopes of the Sierra. I had planned to work another several years and then, simply retire to enjoy my friends here. Perhaps, I would take more extensive trips to the great northern desert, where the pavement ends and the true West begins at the Applegate Trail to Oregon. I would keep eating dinner on Wednesday nights at the Coney Island Bar and Grill. The Prospectors' Club would continue to offer luau parties, cigar, boxing, and drinking night, single malt scotch and fine rum, and poker on Thursday afternoons in the clubroom at Harrah's.

Though I still loved operating, I had become increasingly interested in administrative challenges. I knew that I would do less and less surgery as the years went on, and saw a need to make room for younger people. Our educational program for students and residents was excellent. However, we were faced with a crisis involving the distribution of surgical residents in the statewide training program, which we had initiated in 1980 when Nevadans numbered only about 700,000. Now, there were 1.2 million people in the Las Vegas area and about 350,000 in the rest of the north. I considered an exciting offer to serve Las Vegas veterans at the Nellis Air Force Base Hospital, but their operating room availability was still insufficient. We were doing much more complex surgery on veterans in Northern Nevada, and probably, Washoe Valley will grow to support another surgical arm of the University of Nevada. Yet, Chairman Alex Little recognized what I had known for two decades—with growth, for better or worse, Las Vegas has become the dominant force in Nevada.

In the fall of 1999, during a casual discussion, a senior surgeon in Central Office in Washington, D.C., mentioned the possibility of a position there. In January of 2000, a call came, asking me to fly back to Washington, D.C., for an interview. The committee asked about my successes and also about my failures. I outlined the institutional processes and cultures, including my experience at George Washington, that I regarded to have led to failure and those that I thought led to success. To my pleasure, I was invited to assume the position of national director of surgery for the Veterans Administration. So I planned another 180-degree course change, a return to Washington, D.C., to work in Central Office on Vermont Avenue. This move gave me an enhanced opportunity to continue to care for the "greatest generation" and to the veterans who follow them.

The Department of Veterans Affairs made unparalleled contributions to quality health care and, though we are far from perfect, continues to make innovative organizational contributions. In the past, the question was asked, "What will happen when the 'greatest generation' is gone?" But, in spirit, they will never be gone. Actually, the number of veterans served is increasing, and more new patients appear daily. The reorganized agency had become a model for quality monitoring and quality improvement in health care systems in this country and abroad. It is also not afraid to be self-critical and to continually look at ways to improve. I left the Silver State, with sorrow and fond memories, but I still reach out to it, day after day, and to other hospitals in our system. I find myself now far removed in time and space from the days of "practicing" in the Bronx and Yonkers. Yet, it seems all the same—the same brightness and optimism: practicing and having to learn new things much as in the past. And many challenging things remain to be done.